Systematic screening for active tuberculosis

Principles and recommendations

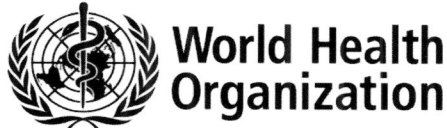

World Health Organization

WHO Library Cataloguing-in-Publication Data

Systematic screening for active tuberculosis: principles and recommendations.

1.Tuberculosis, Multidrug-Resistant - diagnosis. 2.Algorithms. 3.Incidence. 4.Tuberculosis, Multidrug-Resistant - epidemiology. 5.Guideline. I.World Health Organization.

ISBN 978 92 4 154860 1   (NLM classification: WF 220)

Cover design by Dr Knut Lonnroth
Cover image by Kapitza Images

Printed by the WHO Document Production Services, Geneva, Switzerland
WHO/HTM/TB/2013.04

Contents

Supporting material available at : www.who.int/tb/tbscreening
- Systematic reviews
- GRADE summary tables: benefits of screening, by risk group
- Decision tables
- Modelled yield of different algorithms for screening and diagnosis
- Report of the scoping meeting, including PICO questions

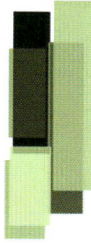

Foreword

Globally, tuberculosis (TB) is a leading cause of death[1] and a major public-health problem.[2] Despite dramatic improvements made since the 1990s in providing access to high-quality TB services,[3] many people with TB remain undiagnosed or are diagnosed only after long delays. The high burden of undiagnosed TB causes much suffering and economic hardship, and sustains transmission.

During the past few years, there has been an intensified discussion about using active case-finding, or screening, as a possible complement to the predominant approach of "passive case-finding". The primary objective of screening is to ensure that active TB is detected early to reduce the risk of poor disease outcomes and the adverse social and economic consequences of the disease, as well as help reduce TB transmission.

There have been calls to revisit the experiences of TB screening campaigns that were widely applied in Europe and North America in the mid-20th century, as well as more recent experiences with TB screening in countries with a high burden of the disease, and to assess their possible relevance for TB care and prevention in the 21st century.

In response, following a thorough review of available evidence WHO has developed guidelines on screening for active TB. The review suggests that screening, if done in the right way and targeting the right people, may reduce suffering and death. However the review also highlights several reasons to be cautious. As discussed in detail in this document, there is a need to balance potential benefits against the risks and costs of screening; this conclusion is mirrored by the history of TB screening.

In 1974, after reviewing the results of several decades of TB screening, the ninth report by WHO's Expert Committee on Tuberculosis recommended that "the policy of indiscriminate tuberculosis case-finding by mobile mass radiography should now be abandoned".[4] Evidence demonstrating the inefficiency of mass screening had mounted, mainly from assessments of populations with a low prevalence of TB and good access to high-quality health services. Mass radiography was expensive, and seemed to add little to what could be achieved through passive case-finding in those settings.[5,6,7] Community screening was deemed inappropriate in low-income settings because basic diagnostic and treatment services were not widely available.[8,9]

WHO has since advised against mass screening. However, there was never an explicit recommendation made against screening as such, and it was never abandoned. "Indiscriminate" is a key word in this rare negative WHO recommendation from 1974, and in fact the report recommended that screening be continued for selected risk groups, such as close contacts of people with TB and immigrants from areas with a high prevalence of the disease.[4] An extensive review of screening experiences in Canada, the former Czechoslovakia and the Netherlands during the 1950s and 1960s, which underpinned WHO's recommendation, concluded that "...radiography might be a more efficient instrument in tuberculosis control, provided that its indiscriminate mass use is replaced by a discriminate one."[5]

Indeed, screening specific risk groups has been part of the *Stop TB strategy* for many years, namely for people living with HIV[10] and household contacts of people with TB.[11] WHO also has guidelines on diagnosing and managing TB in prison populations,[12] in refugees[13] and in people with diabetes,[14] although all of these guidelines contain insufficient advice on how to screen for active TB. Many countries have implemented screening in these risk groups and others, especially low-burden countries that have concentrated epidemics. However during the past few years screening has been implemented in high-burden countries that are striving to close the case-detection gap and reduce the delays in diagnosis that remain a challenge despite scaling up and decentralizing diagnostic and treatment services. The results in these high-burden countries have been mixed, and there are several outstanding questions about the pros and cons of screening.

It makes sense that countries with a low burden of TB that experience an epidemic that is concentrated among specific risk groups – such as immigrants, certain ethnic groups, prisoners, or homeless people – focus their care and prevention efforts particularly on such groups. When resources are available, and when cost-effectiveness is assessed against a range of other expensive health interventions, TB screening in selected risk groups may be affordable and have relatively low opportunity costs. Especially when a country is striving to eliminate TB, and needs to invest additional resources to effectively reach those who are hardest to reach, screening selected high-risk groups may be a key part of the response to TB.[15] But does this strategy make sense in resource-constrained high-burden countries that have a more generalized epidemic? If so, which risk groups should be screened, and what approach should be taken? To answer these questions, one needs to consider the goals of screening, the alternative interventions that can be used to reach those goals, the relative cost-effectiveness of the different approaches, the feasibility and affordability of each approach, and the risk of doing harm through screening – for example, by generating high numbers of false-positive cases.

This document presents the first comprehensive assessment by WHO of the appropriateness of screening for active TB since the recommendations made in 1974 by the Expert Committee. It provides provisional answers to the questions described above. However, the relative effectiveness and cost effectiveness of screening remain uncertain, a point that is underscored by the systematic reviews presented in this guideline. Evidence suggests that some risk groups should always be screened, whereas the prioritization of other risk groups as well as the choice of screening approach depend on the epidemiology, the health-system context, and the resources available.

This document sets out basic principles for prioritizing risk groups and choosing a screening approach. It also emphasizes the importance of assessing the epidemiological situation, adapting approaches to local situations, integrating TB screening into other health-promotion activities, minimizing the risk of harm to individuals, and engaging in continual monitoring and evaluation. It calls for more and better research to assess the impact of screening and to develop and evaluate new screening tests and approaches.

Dr Mario Raviglione
Director, Stop TB Department
World Health Organization

3

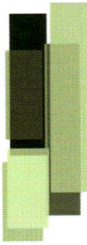

Acknowledgements

The recommendations in this guideline were developed by a Guideline Development Group consisting of the following experts: Dr Sevim Ahmedov (United States Agency for International Development, United States), Dr Helen Ayles (University of Zambia, Zambia), Dr Lucie Blok (KIT Royal Tropical Institute, the Netherlands), Dr Gavin Churchyard (Aurum Institute for Health Research, South Africa), Dr Liz Corbett (MLW Clinical Research Programme, Malawi), Dr Mao Tang Eang (National TB Programme, Cambodia), Dr Peter Godfrey-Faussett (London School of Hygiene and Tropical Medicine, United Kingdom), Dr Jonathan Golub (Johns Hopkins University School of Medicine, United States), Dr Katharina Kranzer (London School of Hygiene and Tropical Medicine, United Kingdom), Dr Josué Lima (National TB Programme, Brazil), Dr Wang Lixia (National TB Programme, People's Republic of China), Dr Thandar Lwin (National TB Programme, Myanmar), Dr Ellen Mitchell (KNCV Tuberculosis Foundation, the Netherlands), Dr Mary Reichler (Centers for Disease Control and Prevention, United States), Dr Adrienne Shapiro (John Hopkins University School of Medicine, United States), Dr Alena Skrahina (National TB Programme, Belarus), Dr Pedro Guillermo Suarez (Management Science for Health, United States), Dr Marieke van der Werf (European Centre for Disease Prevention and Control, Sweden), Dr Anja Van't Hoog (Amsterdam Institute for Global Health and Development, the Netherlands), Dr Norio Yamada (Research Institute for TB, Japan).

Dr David Sinclair (Cochrane Infectious Diseases Group and Liverpool School of Tropical Medicine, United Kingdom) served as the guideline's methodologist.

The WHO steering group consisted of Dr Haileyesus Getahun, Dr Knut Lönnroth, Dr Ikushi Onozaki, Dr Salah Ottmani, Dr Mario Raviglione, Dr Mukund Uplekar, and Ms Diana Weil, from the Stop TB Department, and Mr Jacob Creswell and Dr Suvanand Sahu from the Stop TB Partnership secretariat.

In addition, the following WHO staff contributed to the guideline's development: Dr Leopold Blanc, Dr Daniel Chemtob, Ms Hannah Monica Dias, Dr Dennis Falzon, Dr Philippe Glaziou, Dr Malgosia Grzemska, Mr Wayne Van Gemert and Dr Karin Weyer from the Stop TB Department; Dr Andreas Reis from the Department of Ethics, Equity, Trade and Human Rights; Dr Daniel Kibuga from the Regional Office for Africa; and Dr Catharina van Weezenbeek from the Regional Office for the Western Pacific

The development of the guideline was coordinated by Dr Knut Lönnroth, who also wrote the first draft.

All members of the Guideline Development Group and WHO Secretariat staff involved in developing the guideline reviewed and commented on several iterations of the draft.

Peer review comments on the prefinal draft were received from Dr Martien Borgdorff (University of Amsterdam, the Netherlands), Dr Frank Cobelens (Amsterdam Institute for Global Health and Development, the Netherlands), Dr Paul Douglas (Department of Immigration and Citizenship, Australia), Dr Steven Graham (Childhood TB Subgroup, Centre for International Child Health, Australia), Dr Anthony D Harries (International Union Against Tuberculosis and Lung Disease, United Kingdom), Dr Giovanni B Migliori (European Respiratory Society, WHO Collaborating Centre for TB and Lung Diseases, Italy), Dr Lisa Nelson (WHO HIV Department), and Dr Alasdair Reid (UNAIDS, South Africa).

This guideline was financially supported by the United States Agency for International Development through its consolidated grant and the TB CARE I Collaborative Agreement No. AID-OAA-A-10-0020.

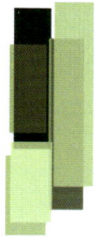

Executive summary

Purpose of the guideline

The purpose of this document is to provide evidence-based:
- key principles to guide the planning and implementation of systematic screening for active tuberculosis (TB);
- recommendations on prioritizing risk groups for systematic screening for active TB; and
- algorithm options for screening and diagnosis of active TB.

The target audience for the guide is principally staff at national TB programmes and other public-health agencies, as well as other public and private partners involved in planning, implementing and monitoring TB-control activities in countries with an intermediate-to-high burden of TB.

Definition of systematic screening for active TB

For the purpose of this guideline, systematic screening for active TB is defined as the *systematic identification of people with suspected active TB, in a predetermined target group, using tests, examinations or other procedures that can be applied rapidly*. The screening tests, examinations or other procedures should efficiently distinguish people with a high probability of having active TB from those who are unlikely to have active TB. Among those whose screening is positive, the diagnosis needs to be established by one or several diagnostic tests and additional clinical assessments, which together have high accuracy.

Systematic screening for active TB is predominantly provider-initiated. It may target people who do not seek health care because they do not have or recognize symptoms, because they do not perceive that they have a health problem that warrants medical attention, because there are barriers to accessing care, or for other reasons. It may also target people seeking health care who do or do not have symptoms or signs compatible with TB and who may not be identified by "passive case-finding" as possibly having TB. People seeking care who may be eligible for TB screening include people with medical conditions that constitute risk factors for TB (such as people living with HIV and people with diabetes mellitus) who may seek care for reasons other than symptoms compatible with TB.

Objectives of systematic screening for active TB

The primary objective of screening for active TB is to ensure that active TB is detected early and treatment is initiated promptly, with the ultimate aim of reducing the risk of poor treatment outcomes, health sequelae and the adverse social and economic consequences of TB, as well as helping to reduce TB transmission.

Reviews of the evidence

In order to develop the principles and recommendations for systematic screening for active TB, WHO established a Guideline Development Group (see Section 4 for information on the guideline development process) and commissioned four systematic reviews (summarized in Section 5; the full reviews can be found under the link "Systematic reviews and PICO questions" available at www.who.int/tb/tbscreening), covering:

- the general benefits of TB screening (Review 1);
- the sensitivity and specificity of different TB screening tools and algorithms (Review 2);
- the number needed to screen to detect one case of active TB in different risk groups (Review 3);
- the acceptability of TB screening in different risk groups (Review 4).

The burden of undetected TB is high in many settings, especially in some risk groups. The delay in diagnosing TB and initiating appropriate treatment is often long, especially in groups with poor access to health care. Many people with active TB do not experience typical TB symptoms in the early stages of the disease. These individuals are unlikely to seek care early, and may not be properly diagnosed when seeking care. Passive case-finding therefore leads to missed or delayed diagnoses for many people. Appropriately diagnosing and treating TB dramatically improves health outcomes when compared with not diagnosing and treating the disease. These observations together constitute indirect evidence that screening for active TB in selected risk groups should benefit individuals and public health.

However, while the systematic reviews show that there is some evidence that screening can improve the early detection of TB, the direct evidence remains weak for the impact of screening on health outcomes and TB transmission when compared with passive case-finding alone. Furthermore, data are lacking on the cost effectiveness of screening compared with other interventions to improve early detection, and it is clear that indiscriminate screening can require a lot of resources.

Therefore, indiscriminate mass screening should be avoided; and screening in selected risk groups requires careful consideration of the potential benefits and risks of harm, including side effects and other harms for the individual from false diagnosis as well as the inappropriate use of health-care resources.

Decisions on when and how to screen for active TB, which risk groups to prioritize and which algorithm to use for screening and diagnosis depend on the epidemiological situation, the capacity of the health system, and the availability of resources.

Key principles for systematic screening for active TB

The following key principles should be considered when planning a TB-screening initiative.

1. *Before screening is initiated, high-quality TB diagnosis, treatment, care, management and support for patients should be in place, and there should be the capacity to scale these up further to match the anticipated rise in case detection that may occur as a result of screening. In addition, a baseline analysis should be completed in order to demonstrate that the potential benefits of screening clearly outweigh the risks of doing harm, and that the required investments in screening are reasonable in relation to the expected benefits.*

2. *Indiscriminate mass screening should be avoided. The prioritization of risk groups for screening should be based on assessments made for each risk group of the potential benefits and harms, the feasibility of the initiative, the acceptability of the approach, the number needed to screen, and the cost effectiveness of screening.*

3. *The choice of algorithm for screening and diagnosis should be based on an assessment of the accuracy of the algorithm for each risk group considered, as well as the availability, feasibility and cost of the tests.*

4. *TB screening should follow established ethical principles for screening for infectious diseases, observe human rights, and be designed to minimize the risk of discomfort, pain, stigma and discrimination.*

5. *The TB screening approach should be developed and implemented in a way that optimizes synergies with the delivery of other health services and social services.*

6. *A screening strategy should be monitored and reassessed continually to inform re-prioritization of risk groups, re-adaptation of screening approaches when necessary and discontinuation of screening at an appropriate time.*

Details on the key principles are provided in Section 7.

Recommendations on risk groups to screen

Seven recommendations on prioritizing risk groups for screening have been developed. The recommendations are divided into strong recommendations and conditional recommendations.

A **strong recommendation** is one for which the desirable effects of adhering to the recommendation are judged to clearly outweigh the undesirable effects, and for which screening is judged to be feasible, acceptable and affordable in all settings.

A **conditional recommendation** is one for which the desirable effects of adhering to the recommendation probably outweigh the undesirable effects but the trade-offs, cost effectiveness, feasibility or affordability, or some combination of these, are uncertain. Reasons for uncertainty may include:

- a lack of high-quality evidence to support the recommendation;
- evidence of limited benefits from implementing the recommendation;
- high costs or low feasibility or acceptability, or a combination of these.

Recommendations have not been developed for all of the risk groups initially considered due to a lack of evidence; in particular in Review 1 (the systematic review of the general benefits of screening) there was a lack of studies assessing outcomes judged to be critical for several risk groups (see Sections 4.2 and 5). Additional risk groups may be considered for screening based on the criteria set out in the key principles in Section 7.

The recommendations are listed below. For details on the evidence, see Section 5 and *Annex I* in this document, and supporting at www.who.int/tb/tbscreening. See Section 8 in this document for remarks on each recommendation.

Strong recommendations
<u>Recommendation 1:</u> *Household contacts and other close contacts should be systematically screened for active TB.*

<u>Recommendation 2:</u> *People living with HIV should be systematically screened for active TB at each visit to a health facility.*

<u>Recommendation 3:</u> *Current and former workers in workplaces with silica exposure should be systematically screened for active TB.*

Conditional recommendations
<u>Recommendation 4:</u> *Systematic screening for active TB should be considered in prisons and other penitentiary institutions.*

<u>Recommendation 5:</u> *Systematic screening for active TB should be considered in people with an untreated fibrotic chest X-ray lesion.*

<u>Recommendation 6:</u> *In settings where the TB prevalence in the general population is 100/100 000 population or higher, systematic screening for active TB should be considered among people who are seeking health care or* **11** *who are in health care and who belong to selected risk groups. (The risk*

groups to be considered are listed in the remarks to this recommendation in Section 8).

Recommendation 7:
(a) Systematic screening for active TB may be considered for geographically defined subpopulations with extremely high levels of undetected TB (1% prevalence or higher).
(b) Systematic screening for active TB may be considered also for other subpopulations that have very poor access to health care, such as people living in urban slums, homeless people, people living in remote areas with poor access to health care, and other vulnerable or marginalized groups including some indigenous populations, migrants and refugees.

Algorithms for screening and diagnosis

Different screening algorithm options have been developed for adults and children. (See Section 5.2 for a summary of the evidence, Section 9 for remarks on each algorithm, and *Annex II* and *Annex III* in this document, as well as supporting material available at www.who.int/tb/tbscreening for details on the accuracy of different tests, the flow charts of the algorithms and the modelled yield for each algorithm for adults.)

Options for the initial screening include screening for symptoms (screening either for cough lasting for longer than 2 weeks, or screening for any symptom compatible with TB, including cough of any duration, haemoptysis, weight loss, fever or night sweats) or screening with chest radiography. If symptom screening is used initially, then chest radiography can be used as a second screen to improve the pretest probability of the subsequent diagnostic test, and to reduce the number of people who need to undergo further diagnostic evaluation.

As part of the initial screening, each algorithm includes steps to identify people living with HIV; these persons should be screened and diagnosed by following the algorithm for people living with HIV in *Guidelines for intensified tuberculosis case-finding and isoniazid preventive therapy for people living with HIV in resource-constrained settings.*[10] Screening can therefore be enhanced by combining screening for TB with screening for HIV.

Each algorithm for adults includes options for the initial diagnostic testing of people whose screening test is positive: either sputum-smear microscopy[i] or a rapid molecular test that has been demonstrated to have high accuracy for both smear-positive and smear-negative pulmonary TB, such as the Xpert MTB/RIF test (Cepheid, Sunnyvale, CA) (or any rapid test recommended by WHO in the future and that has the same or better accuracy). Positive or negative diagnostic results may require a repeat test or further diagnostic evaluation using culture, drug-susceptibility testing, clinical assessment, or some combination of these. Culture is the gold standard of diagnostic testing for TB. However, in these algorithms it is not considered for use as an initial diagnostic test because it demands more resources and requires a much longer wait for results (2–6 weeks) than both the Xpert MTB/RIF test and sputum-smear microscopy, both of which can provide final test results in less than 1 day. Where resources permit, and where the health system has sufficient capacity to ensure that patients are followed up after culture results are available, culture may be used in parallel with or after testing with the Xpert MTB/RIF or sputum-smear microscopy. Culture with drug-susceptibility testing should be done according to guidelines for diagnosing drug-resistant TB.[16]

The algorithms have been developed predominantly to detect pulmonary TB. The accuracy of tests for screening and diagnosis has been assessed using culture-confirmed pulmonary TB as the gold standard.

The algorithms all have different sensitivity and specificity (see Section 5.2), and therefore different yields of true-positive and true-negative cases and false-positive and false-negative TB. Yields also vary with TB prevalence in the screened population. For all algorithms, the risk of a false-positive diagnosis increases as the prevalence declines; therefore, special attention must be paid to diagnostic accuracy, particularly when the prevalence of TB in the screened population is less than 1%.

The algorithms have different costs, and requirements in terms of human resources and health systems. The choice of algorithm for screening and diagnosis depends on the risk group, the prevalence of TB, the availability of

---

[i] This refers to conventional light microscopy used to examine direct smears stained with Ziehl–Neelsen (with or without specific sputum-processing methods) or fluorescence microscopy (including microscopy with light-emitting diodes).

resources and feasibility. See Section 8 for remarks about choosing an appropriate algorithm for different risk groups.

The algorithms are described below.

Screening in adults and children aged 10 years or older

Option 1: This algorithm includes an interview about TB symptoms and HIV status. All people with cough lasting longer than 2 weeks should be investigated for TB. Chest radiography should be considered as a second screening for people who have had cough lasting longer than 2 weeks; people with an abnormal chest radiograph suggestive of TB[ii] should be evaluated for TB. For people known to be HIV-positive, see the Guidelines for intensified tuberculosis case-finding and isoniazid preventive therapy for people living with HIV in resource-constrained settings.[10]

Option 2: This algorithm includes an interview about TB symptoms and HIV status. Further investigation for TB should be done for persons with any of the following symptoms: cough of any duration, haemoptysis, weight loss, fever or night sweats. Chest radiography should be considered as a second screening for people who screened positive when asked about symptoms; and people with an abnormal chest radiograph suggestive of TB should be evaluated for TB. For persons known to be HIV-positive, see the Guidelines for intensified tuberculosis case-finding and isoniazid preventive therapy for people living with HIV in resource-constrained settings.[10]

Option 3: This algorithm includes chest radiography and an interview about HIV status. Persons with an abnormal chest radiograph suggestive of TB should be evaluated for TB. For persons known to be HIV-positive, see the Guidelines for intensified tuberculosis case-finding and isoniazid preventive therapy for people living with HIV in resource-constrained settings .[10]

[ii] Chest radiographs suggestive of TB may be separated into those that are suggestive of active TB, and those that are suggestive of either active or inactive TB (see Section 9 for details).

Screening in children aged younger than 10 years

Screening children who are living with HIV or who are contacts of someone with TB

- For children who are living with HIV or who are contacts of someone with TB, symptom-based screening should be done to identify those with cough, fever, weight loss or fatigue of any duration; children with any symptom should be investigated for TB.
- For children who are living with HIV or who are contacts of someone with TB, chest radiography may be added to the initial screening. Children with any symptom or a chest radiograph with an abnormality suggestive of TB should be investigated for TB.

Screening children in situations other than as part of contact investigation or screening among people living with HIV

- For children who are younger than 10 years and who are screened in situations other than as part of contact investigation or screening for people living with HIV, an interview should be done to determine whether the child is known to be HIV-positive or has had recent contact with someone who has TB, in either case the algorithm options for children younger than 10 years who are living with HIV or who are contacts of someone with TB apply.

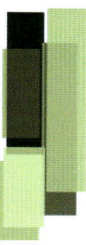

Abbreviations

GRADE   Grading of Recommendations Assessment, Development and Evaluation

MDR-TB   Multidrug-resistant TB

NNS   Number needed to screen (to detect one case of active tuberculosis)

NPV   Negative predictive value

PPV   Positive predictive value

PTP   Pretest probability

TB   Tuberculosis

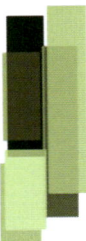

Definitions

Active tuberculosis
Active tuberculosis refers to disease that occurs in someone infected with *Mycobacterium tuberculosis*. It is characterized by signs or symptoms of active disease, or both, and is distinct from latent tuberculosis infection, which occurs without signs or symptoms of active disease.

Active tuberculosis case-finding
Active case-finding is synonymous with systematic screening for active TB, although it normally implies screening that is implemented outside of health facilities.

Enhanced tuberculosis case-finding
Enhanced case-finding uses health information or education to provide information about what type of health-seeking behaviour is appropriate when people experience symptoms of TB; this type of case-finding may be combined with improving access to diagnostic services. Enhanced case-finding may or may not be combined with screening.

Initial screening
The first screening test, examination or other procedure applied in the population eligible for screening.

Number needed to screen
The number needed to screen is the number of persons that need to undergo screening in order to diagnose one person with active TB.

Passive tuberculosis case-finding
A patient-initiated pathway to TB diagnosis involving: (1) a person with active TB experiencing symptoms that he or she recognizes as serious; (2) the person having access to and seeking care, and presenting spontaneously at an appropriate health facility; (3) a health worker correctly assessing whether the person fulfils the criteria for suspected TB; and (4) the successful use of a diagnostic algorithm with sufficient sensitivity and

specificity. Passive case-finding may involve an element of systematic screening if the identification of people with suspected TB is done systematically for all people seeking care in a health facility or clinic.

Repeat screening
Rescreening in the same population at a given interval.

Risk groups
A risk group is any group of people in which the prevalence or incidence of TB is significantly higher than in the general population.

Screening test, examination or procedure for active tuberculosis
A test, examination or other procedure for active tuberculosis distinguishes people with a high likelihood of having active TB from people who are highly unlikely to have active TB. A screening test is not intended to be diagnostic. People with positive results on a screening test should undergo diagnostic evaluation.

Second screening
A second screening test, examination or other procedure applied to persons whose results were positive during the initial screen.

Systematic screening for active TB
Systematic screening for active TB is the systematic identification of people with suspected active TB, in a predetermined target group, using tests, examinations or other procedures that can be applied rapidly. Among those screened positive, the diagnosis needs to be established by one or several diagnostic tests and additional clinical assessments, which together have high accuracy.

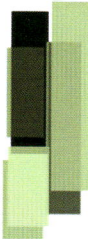

1. Purpose of guideline and target audience

1.1 Purpose

This document provides evidence-based:
1. key principles to guide the planning and implementation of systematic screening for active tuberculosis (TB);
2. recommendations on prioritizing risk groups for systematic screening for active TB;
3. algorithm options for screening and diagnosis.

Guidelines are already available for screening for TB in people living with HIV[10] and for contact investigation.[11] There are also guidelines on caring for people with TB and preventing TB in prisons,[12] among refugees and displaced populations,[13] among intravenous drug users and other drug users,[17] and in people with diabetes;[14] all of these guidelines also address the early detection of TB. There is also extensive guidance on diagnosing TB (see http://www.who.int/tb/laboratory/tool_set/en/index.html). This document refers to the guidelines described above and others, when appropriate.

Manuals and tools for how to plan and implement screening in specific risk groups are not included in this document but will be provided in subsequent publications.

This guideline does not specifically address screening for latent TB infection, although it will highlight how ruling out active TB can help identify people eligible for treatment for latent infection.

1.2 Target audience

The guideline principally targets countries with an intermediate-to-high burden of TB.

The main target audience is the staff of national TB programmes and other public-health agencies, and other public and private health-care providers and organizations involved in planning, implementing and monitoring TB care and prevention activities. The principles and recommendations are also relevant to health-care staff. However, specific operational guidance is not included in this document. Moreover, the recommendations provided here must be adapted to local settings. National and subnational recommendations must be developed by national TB programmes and other national and subnational public-health agencies and partners; recommendations developed by national and subnational agencies should guide health-care staff in specific settings.

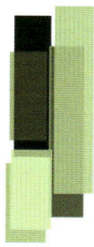

2. Definition of screening for active TB in risk groups

2.1 Systematic screening for active TB

In this guideline, systematic screening for active TB is defined as the *systematic identification of people with suspected active TB, in a predetermined target group, using tests, examinations or other procedures that can be applied rapidly.*

The screening tests, examinations or other procedures should efficiently distinguish persons with a high probability of having TB (that is, with suspected TB) from those who are unlikely to have TB. Among those whose screening is positive, the diagnosis needs to be established by using one or several diagnostic tests and additional clinical assessments, which together have high accuracy.

In principle, systematic screening for active TB can be done for the whole population (mass screening) or be targeted at selected risk groups. It can target people who seek health care (with or without symptoms or signs compatible with TB) and people who do not seek care (because they do not perceive that they have a health problem that warrants medical attention, because barriers make it difficult to access health care, or for other reasons).

Passive case-finding can be complemented by screening – for example, if all people seeking care are systematically asked about TB symptoms. Therefore, screening and passive case-finding are not mutually exclusive. In principle, screening is provider-initiated, and offered to a predetermined target group. However, once a screening test is made available, it may be requested by people who want to be screened. The term active case-finding is often used synonymously with screening, although it usually implies screening that is offered outside of health facilities.[18]

23

2.2 Risk groups

A risk group for TB is any group of people within which the prevalence or incidence of TB is significantly higher than in the general population. A risk group may be a group of people sharing a specific individual-level risk profile (for example, being in close contact with a person who has active TB; or living with HIV or having diabetes; or being a migrant). A risk group can also be defined as all people living in a specific geographical location associated with a high burden of TB (for example, all people living in an urban slum) or a specific type of institution (such as all prisoners in a country).

It is not necessary that the characterizing factor is a causal risk factor for TB. The association of a risk marker with TB may be confounded by other factors, but it is still valid as an identifier for having a high risk of TB.

An absolute level of TB prevalence or incidence may be used as a cut-off to define a risk group in a given epidemiological situation. For example, in Europe, where TB notification often is a good estimate of TB incidence, risk groups have been defined as those in which TB notification is more than 100/100 000[15] population, which is considerably higher than the incidence in the general population in the region. In the Netherlands, the cut-off was set at more than 50/100 000 population, since this was about 10 times the national average.[19] Any absolute level must be adapted to the local situation, and it may also change over time as the burden and distribution of TB change.

For practical purposes, it may be useful to categorize risk groups according to the places where they can be reached for screening. *Table 1* lists risk groups that may be considered, and attempts to categorize them. The list is not exhaustive and risk groups may be reachable in different places depending on the local epidemiological situation and health-system context.

Table 1. **Possible risk groups to consider for screening for tuberculosis**

Potential site of screening	Risk group
Community	Geographical areas with a high prevalence
	Subpopulations with poor access to health care and with other associated risk factors (such as living in a poor area, an urban slum or a remote area; being a member of an indigenous or tribal population, or a migrant, refugee, homeless, or nomadic; being a sex worker)
Hospital outpatient and inpatient departments, and primary health-care centres	People previously treated for TB
	People with an untreated fibrotic lesion identified by chest radiography
	People living with HIV and people attending HIV testing
	People with diabetes mellitus
	People with chronic respiratory disease and smokers
	Undernourished people
	People with gastrectomy or jejunoileal bypass
	People with an alcohol-use disorder and intravenous drug users
	People with chronic renal failure
	People having treatments that compromise their immune system
	Elderly people
	People in mental health clinics or institutions
Residential institutions	Prisoners and prison staff
	People residing in shelters
	Other congregate institutions (such as the military)
Immigration and refugee services	Immigrants from settings with a high prevalence of TB
	People in refugee camps
Workplaces	Health-care workers
	Miners or others who are exposed to silica
	Other workplaces with a high prevalence of TB

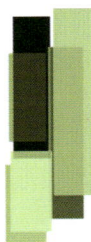

3. Rationale and objectives of screening for active TB

3.1 Challenges to TB care and control

Large pool of undetected TB
The global prevalence of TB and death rates from the disease are steadily declining.[3] The scaling up of high-quality diagnosis and treatment of TB have greatly contributed to these reductions by improving cure rates and reducing case–fatality rates.[20] Still, in 2011, 8.7 million people developed TB and 1.4 million people died from the disease. Moreover, the estimated global incidence of TB is declining slowly, by less than 2% per year. To reach the TB elimination target of less than 1 case/1 000 000 population in 2050, the incidence needs to decline by 20% per year.[3]

Missed diagnoses or delayed diagnoses, and problems with access to high-quality care lead to a higher risk of death, suffering, sequelae and catastrophic financial consequences. These missed opportunities also lead to a longer duration of infectiousness for individuals, and thus sustain transmission,[21,22,23] especially where population density is high and where living and working conditions are poor, including conditions that are overcrowded and have inadequate ventilation.[24]

WHO estimates that about one third of all incident cases of active TB are not properly diagnosed or receive care of questionable quality outside of national TB programmes and are not being notified.[3] Among those cases who are eventually diagnosed, the delay is often long.[25,26] There is abundant direct evidence from national surveys of TB prevalence[27,28,29] and other research[30] that the pool of undetected TB cases remains large in many countries despite the scaling up and decentralizing of TB diagnosis and treatment, particularly in certain risk groups, such as people living with HIV,[31] close contacts of people with TB,[32,33] miners,[30,34] prisoners,[35] homeless people,[36] and several clinical risk groups.[30]

Children with TB are likely to represent a large proportion of the pool of undetected TB, but the size of the proportion is uncertain.[37] This is particularly the case for young children, for whom clinical overlap is common between the features of childhood TB and other frequent and often fatal causes of mortality among children younger than 5 years, such as pneumonia, malnutrition, meningitis and HIV. The prevalence of TB disease among children who are close contacts of a TB case is high.[32,33] Therefore, screening children who are contacts is already widely recommended, although it is rarely implemented systematically.[38,39]

Limitations of passive case-finding using sputum-smear microscopy
Passive case-finding (that is, identifying TB among people who are actively seeking care)[40] with diagnosis based mainly on sputum-smear microscopy is effective in diagnosing highly infectious TB (that is, sputum smear-positive TB in a person with a productive cough), but it is less effective in early diagnosis for people with less pronounced symptoms. Since early 2000, all surveys of TB prevalence done in countries with reasonably well performing national TB programmes have consistently demonstrated that the majority of undiagnosed cases of pulmonary TB are sputum-smear negative. They have also demonstrated that more than 50% of those with prevalent bacteriologically confirmed pulmonary TB do not report symptoms that correspond to the commonly used criteria for suspecting disease and prompting diagnostic investigation (that is, cough lasting longer than 2–3 weeks); additionally, a large proportion of these cases do not report any symptoms at all.[27,28,29] These individuals are less likely to seek care than people with more prominent symptoms. When they do seek care, they are less likely to be diagnosed.

These observation are not new, and are to be expected when the priority is to detect the most infectious cases. An anticipated result of effective diagnosis and treatment that uses passive case-finding to identify smear-positive cases is that the proportion of smear-positive cases with chronic cough in the total prevalence pool will gradually diminish; this has been demonstrated by findings from repeated prevalence surveys in China.[41] Smear-positive TB with productive cough is associated with a rate of transmission that is four to five times higher than that for smear-negative pulmonary TB.[42,43] However, as the proportion of cases with smear-negative culture-positive TB increases among the prevalent cases of pulmonary TB in the community, the relative contribution of these cases to the total burden of TB and to total transmission will gradually increase, although the contribution of smear-negative TB to total transmission will probably not be above 15–20%.[42,43]

When case detection is high and the success rate for treating smear-positive cases with chronic cough is also high, further actions to improve passive case-finding are unlikely to have an increased impact on transmission unless additional efforts are put in place to detect both smear-positive and smear-negative cases early.[44] Screening for active TB is one of several possible interventions that can improve early detection of all forms of TB, but providing better access to diagnostic tests that are more sensitive than smear microscopy is the first essential step.

Reaching the poorest people more effectively
Passive case-finding relies on four actions: (1) a person with active TB experiencing and recognizing symptoms, (2) the person presenting to an appropriate health facility, (3) a health-worker correctly assessing whether the person fulfils the criteria for suspected TB, and (4) the successful application of a complete diagnostic algorithm with sufficient sensitivity and specificity.[45] Barriers to early case detection may occur at each step, and the poorest people are at highest risk of not completing, or delaying, each step. They have the least access to high-quality services, and face the highest costs from illness and for health care.[24] Screening groups who have limited access to health care may help reduce delays. However, other interventions to improve health-seeking and access may be equally or more relevant and cost effective, depending on the local situation.

Detecting TB early in other vulnerable groups
People living with HIV, young children, elderly people, people with diabetes, and other groups who have compromised immune systems face a high risk of poor outcomes from TB treatment, including relapse and death. The risk is augmented when diagnosis is delayed. Systematic screening can be particularly beneficial for these groups. However, the first essential action is to ensure that diagnostic procedures are optimal among people actively seeking care.

3.2 Objectives and goals of screening for active TB

The *primary objective* of screening is to detect active TB early; this can contribute to two ultimate goals:
1. reducing the risk of poor treatment outcomes, health sequelae, and the adverse social and economic consequences of TB for the individual. This reduces suffering, the prevalence of TB, and death from TB;
2. reducing TB transmission by shortening of the duration of infectiousness. This reduces the incidence of TB infection and consequently contributes to reduced incidence of TB disease.

A *second objective* is to rule out active disease to help identify people who are eligible for treatment of latent TB infection – for example, among people living with HIV and contacts who are younger than 5 years.

Furthermore, screening can help identify people who are at particularly high risk of developing active disease in the future and thus may require repeat screening; for example, this group includes people with an abnormal chest radiograph that is compatible with TB but who were not diagnosed with active disease at the time of screening.

Combining screening for TB with screening for TB risk factors can also help map individual or community-level risk factors and socioeconomic determinants that need to be addressed to more effectively prevent the disease.

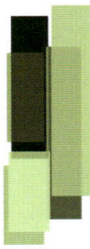

4. Guideline development process

4.1 Scoping, Guideline Development Group and peer review

A scoping meeting was organized by WHO in June 2011[46] to assess the need to develop guidelines on TB screening, to scope the evidence, identify key research questions and related knowledge gaps, define PICO questions and develop a plan of work, including establishing a steering group and a Guideline Development Group. After an open call for applications, four systematic reviews were subsequently commissioned on:

- the general benefits of TB screening (Review 1);
- the sensitivity and specificity of different screening tools and algorithms (Review 2);
- the number needed to screen to detect one case of TB in different risk groups (Review 3);
- the acceptability of screening in different risk groups (Review 4).

The PICO questions for each review and the systematic reviews are available as supporting material in the folder "Systematic reviews and PICO questions" at www.who.int/tb/tbscreening.

A meeting to review the data was organized for June 2012, at the time when three systematic reviews had been almost finalized, and one review had just started. At that meeting preliminary findings were discussed, and a plan was developed to complete the final analyses before the final guideline meeting.

The final guideline meeting was convened in October 2012. Ahead of the meeting, the final reports of the systematic reviews, the tables showing the Grading of Recommendations Assessment, Development and Evaluation (the GRADE tables) and the Decision tables (see below) were circulated to members. Each Decision table and its related GRADE tables were discussed separately, and the guideline group either developed recommendations or decided that there was insufficient evidence to develop a recommendation.

Consensus was sought for each recommendation, and all members of the group were asked if they agreed with the final recommendation. When consensus was not reached, different options for the recommendation were drafted and voted on; divergent opinions were recorded. Voting was necessary for only one recommendation (see Section 8).

Draft guidelines were circulated to a group of peer reviewers, consisting of all staff of the Stop TB Department at WHO's headquarters and staff of other selected departments, regional TB advisers, managers of selected national TB programmes, other national stakeholders involved in TB care and control in selected countries, working groups in the Stop TB Partnership, organizations providing technical support to TB care and control activities, and individuals with expertise in TB care and control (see *Annex IV*).

The group's work was coordinated with the group developing guidelines on investigating contacts of people with TB.[11] Some of the databases for the systematic reviews were shared. Consistency and cross-referencing between the two guidelines has been ensured.

The members of the Guideline Development Group and persons who provided specific feedback during the peer-review process are listed in *Annex IV*. Conflict–of-interest forms were collected from all members before each meeting, and from peer reviewers who provided comments. None of the experts declared any conflicts of interest that were judged to significantly affect the development of the guideline.

Funds for the development of the guideline were contributed by the United States Agency for International Development through the TB CARE mechanism (grant TB CARE APA2, C1.12).

4.2 GRADE tables and Decision tables

GRADE tables were prepared for all PICO questions addressed by Reviews 1 and 2.

Review 1 (the general benefits of TB screening)
For Review 1, a summary GRADE table was first developed to analyse the evidence for each PICO question across all risk groups combined (see *Annex I*)

then additional tables were developed separately for each risk group for which there was sufficient evidence; the risk groups were close contacts of someone with TB, people living with HIV, prisoners, miners, people with an untreated fibrotic lesion identified by chest radiography, people in high-risk communities and homeless people (for additional information, see supporting material at www.who.int/tb/tbscreening).

The outcomes judged to be critical for Review 1 were: TB case detection if assessed in a controlled trial, outcomes from TB treatment, and the prevalence or incidence of TB. The following outcomes were judged to be important but not critical: the contribution to case detection made by screening measured as a proportion of the total cases detected, the time to diagnosis, and signs of severe disease at time of diagnosis.

Decision tables were developed for each risk group for which published studies were included in Review 1. In addition, a combined Decision table was prepared for people seeking health care who belonged to any of the following risk groups: undernourished people, smokers, people with chronic obstructive pulmonary disease, people with diabetes, people with alcohol-use or substance-use disorders, people with diseases or undergoing treatments that compromise their immune system, people older than 60 years, and pregnant women.

Each Decision table includes background information on the burden of TB, risk of poor treatment results, information on the accuracy of tests for screening and diagnosis, the potential benefits and harms of screening, and information on costs and cost effectiveness (see supporting material at www.who.int/tb/tbscreening.

There were insufficient data to develop separate Decision tables for health-care workers, people who had been previously treated for TB, and migrants. No studies in Review 1 assessed the outcomes judged to be critical for these risk groups. Screening for active TB in people previously treated for TB and in health-care workers has been included as part of screening within health-care facilities (Recommendation 6 in Section 8.2). Migrants, including refugees and immigrants from high-burden settings, are considered as part of community screening (Recommendation 7 in Section 8.2).

Visa applicants from a high-burden country seeking to move to a low-burden country comprise a special category: they may be considered to be a member of a high-risk group by the country to which they are moving but normally they are not considered to be a member of a high-risk group in their country of origin. Review 1 did not include any study assessing the critical outcomes for this risk group. No specific recommendations have been developed for this group.

Review 2 (the sensitivity and specificity of different screening tools and algorithms)

GRADE tables were also developed for the evidence from Review 2 using the modified Quality Assessment of Diagnostic Accuracy Studies (QUADAS-2) instrument[47,48] (see *Annex II*). The algorithms for screening and diagnosis were developed using the GRADE tables and the modelled yield of different algorithms at different levels of TB prevalence (which was based on estimates of screening-test accuracy as well as estimates of the accuracy of diagnostic tests, see Section 5.2 and *Annex II* in this document, and supporting material available at www.who.int/tb/tbscreening).

Review 3 (the number needed to screen to detect one case of TB in different risk groups) and Review 4 (the acceptability of screening in different risk groups)

Review 3 and Review 4 did not assess the effectiveness of interventions or the accuracy of tests, and so were considered to provide background information for the recommendations. No GRADE tables were developed for the evidence from these reviews.

4.3   Grading the recommendations

Recommendations on the specific risk groups that should be considered for screening were graded as *strong* or *conditional*. The grading of the recommendations was based on:
- the strength of the direct evidence of benefit compared with the harms of screening in a given risk group;
- indirect evidence of the benefit of screening, including evidence on the burden of undiagnosed TB in a given risk group and evidence of the risk of poor health outcomes in the absence of treatment or caused by delays in diagnosis and treatment;

- the feasibility, acceptability and cost implications of screening, including the possibility of efficiently identifying and reaching people in a given risk group without violating basic ethical principles.

A **strong recommendation** is one for which the desirable effects of adhering to the recommendation are judged to clearly outweigh the undesirable effects, and for which screening is judged to be feasible, acceptable and affordable in all settings.

A **conditional recommendation** is one for which the desirable effects of adhering to the recommendation probably outweigh the undesirable effects, but the trade-offs, cost effectiveness, feasibility or affordability, or some combination of these, are uncertain. Reasons for uncertainty may include:
- a lack of high-quality evidence to support the recommendation;
- evidence of limited benefits from implementing the recommendation;
- high costs, or low feasibility or acceptability, or a combination of these.

The degree of uncertainty about the trade-offs between the desirable effects and undesirable effects of following each of the conditional recommendations varies across settings, depending on the epidemiological situation and the health system. Therefore, in this guideline, a conditional recommendation implies that:
- the appropriateness of adhering to the recommendation needs to be assessed in each setting; and
- there is a need to prioritize risk groups for screening in each setting.

The overall quality of the direct evidence of benefit compared with evidence of harm ranged from very low to low for all risk groups considered (see Section 5). The values and preferences of the members of the guideline development group therefore significantly influenced the interpretation of indirect evidence and the grading of the recommendations.

The Guideline Development Group placed high value on ensuring that TB is diagnosed early in groups that have a particularly high likelihood of undetected TB and a high risk of poor health outcomes in the absence of early diagnosis and treatment, even if direct evidence of benefit from screening was lacking. Therefore, strong recommendations have been made despite the lack of high-quality direct evidence for three risk groups.

However, the Guideline Development Group also strongly emphasized the need for careful prioritization that considers the opportunity costs of screening, both across risk groups and in relation to other interventions aimed at improving early diagnosis, treatment and prevention. Therefore, owing to the lack of high-quality direct evidence comparing benefits with harms and on the cost effectiveness of screening, the majority of the recommendations made about screening specific risk groups are conditional. Furthermore, the Guideline Development Group emphasized the importance of avoiding the risk of doing harm through screening – that is, both harm to the screened individual and indirect harm by misusing health resources. While the Guideline Development Group did not make any specific negative recommendations (that is, recommendations not to screen in certain situations), the group agreed that a key principle is to avoid indiscriminate screening, and that risk groups should be carefully prioritized for screening using set criteria (outlined in Section 7.2).

Graded recommendations have not been made on which algorithms should be used for screening and diagnosing TB in specific risk groups. Instead, options for screening and diagnosis have been developed; these are presented with remarks about the key issues that should be considered when choosing algorithms for different risk groups, and different epidemiological situations and health systems.

4.4 Proposed subsidiary guideline products and implementation plan

All of the partners included in the guideline-development process have a wide network of experts in different areas and countries who provide technical assistance to national TB control programmes and other country partners engaged in TB care and control; these experts can help with local adaptation of the recommendations and algorithm options. The guideline will be widely disseminated, as will technical assistance from WHO and its partners, to help adapt the guideline to local situations and to mobilize resources.

The impact of the guideline should be evaluated by collecting data from the routine operation of TB surveillance systems (that is, by monitoring case detection, and using disaggregated data on the source of detection and type of case-finding strategy) and through operational research.

Practical tools for assessing the TB situation, prioritizing risk groups and creating national screening strategies for TB will be developed during 2013–2014.

These guidelines are anticipated to need revision within 5 years from their completion; the revision will use additional evidence and lessons learnt from field implementation.

The Guideline Development Group advised WHO to stimulate and coordinate research, and develop guidelines on:
- screening, diagnosing and treating latent TB infection;
- screening for active and latent TB in health-care workers;
- screening for active and latent TB in immigrants from high-prevalence countries.

5. Summaries of the systematic reviews

5.1 Review 1: systematic review of the benefits of systematic screening for active TB to communities and individuals

This review included 61 studies addressing one or several of the study questions for one or several risk groups. (The full review is available in the supporting material at www.who.int/tb/tbscreening) *Annex I* provides a summary GRADE table of the evidence for all risk groups combined. GRADE tables and related Decision tables for each risk group are shown in the supporting material on the Internet. Findings across all risk groups are summarized below. Full references for the studies cited are available in the supporting material on the Internet.

Question 1. When compared with passive case-finding alone does TB screening increase the number of TB cases detected?
The evidence ranges from very low quality to low quality that screening may increase the number of cases found in the short term; the medium-term and long-term effects are unclear. The extent of the increase in the number of cases detected seems to depend on which risk group is screened, the size of the risk group, and the methods used. When a diagnostic algorithm is used that is more sensitive than the algorithm used in passive case-finding, the increase in the number of cases may result from the difference in the diagnostic algorithm rather than from the screening approach itself. Details are provided in *Box 1*.

Box 1. Detailed findings for question 1: When compared with passive case-finding alone does TB screening increase the number of TB cases detected?

Data from 18 prevalence surveys demonstrated that in many settings more than half of the prevalent TB cases in a community are undiagnosed. Screening programmes targeting entire communities through mass screening, or targeting a combination of risk groups (such as combinations of current and former prisoners, people who are HIV-positive, people who are socioeconomically vulnerable, people living in shelters or orphanages, people attending support groups for alcohol users, and people who attend a clinic regularly for follow up of a known lesion seen on chest X-ray), may account for a high proportion of all notified cases in the targeted area. In six studies using mass screening or targeting combinations of risk groups the proportions that these groups accounted for ranged from 18% to 85% of the total number of cases (Meijer 1971, Krivinka 1974, Aneja 1981, Santha 2003, Gonzales-Ochoa 2009, Garcia-Garcia 2000). Targeting a single risk group that has a very high risk of TB seems to contribute fewer cases. For example, screening contacts contributed between 1% and 9% of adult cases in five studies (Capewell 1974, Ormerod 1993, Jereb 1999, Lee 2008, Ottmani 2009). One study targeting only centres that provide voluntary counselling and testing for HIV identified 1% of all cases in an urban area in India (Shetty 2008). One study of screening in drug users and homeless persons in the Netherlands identified 5% of all notified cases (de Vries 2007).

From the above studies it is not possible to confidently conclude whether screening contributed additional cases or only identified cases that would have been detected through passive case-finding, possibly after a longer delay. For such an evaluation, a controlled design comparing areas with and without screening is required. Five randomized controlled trials were identified that investigated the effect of screening on TB case-finding over a short period. They compared TB case-notification rates among communities or individuals. In Brazil, door-to-door screening increased the case yield during the intervention (six months) but not overall during the entire follow-up period of the study (eight months); thus the effect seemed to reduce delay rather than reduce the total number of people diagnosed (Miller 2010). Two Ethiopian studies used community health workers in different ways to increase case-finding and diagnosis. One of the studies used preadvertised outreach clinics (Shargie 2006), and the other implemented activities to increase awareness of TB and TB symptoms, facilitate sputum collection in the community, and support treatment (Datiko 2009). Both found higher case-detection rates in the intervention communities, although the difference was not statistically significant in one study. A South African study followed a cohort of infants randomized to household screening or passive case-finding, and found that screening increased case notification (Moyo 2012). A large trial in South Africa and Zambia did not find any difference in case notification over 3 years; the study compared standard case-findings practices with a package of repeated information campaigns about TB aimed at the community, decentralized sputum collection points with easy access, and sputum collection in health camps (Ayles 2012). While these trials were generally of high quality, the results cannot be generalized with confidence because there were few trials, and each used different screening approaches; they were carried out in a limited number of settings; results were not consistent; and most assessed the impact over only a short time.

Note: *Full references for the studies cited are available in the supporting material on the Internet.*

Question 2. *Compared with passive case-finding does TB screening among people with active TB identify cases at an earlier stage of disease?*

The evidence ranges from very low quality to low quality that screening identifies cases earlier and with less severe disease than passive case-finding does. This may be partly attributed to screening studies using more sensitive diagnostic methods than routine programmes. It may also be due to length–time bias by which people with less severe disease that progresses more slowly are relatively more likely to be detected through screening than people with disease that progresses rapidly. However, early detection of slowly progressing disease may be an objective of screening. Details are provided in *Box 2*.

Box 2. **Detailed findings for question 2: Compared with passive case-finding does TB screening among people with active TB identify cases at an earlier stage of disease?**

All studies that reported the proportion of cases with smear-positive disease among screened cases compared with passively detected cases found that those who were identified through screening were less likely to be smear-positive (Meijer 1971, Krivinka 1974, Ross 1977, Capewell 1986, LeBue 2004, den Boon 2008, Shetty 2008, Story 2008, , Eang 2012,). This would be expected if smear testing were the primary method used in routine diagnosis for passive case-finding, as was the case in South Africa (den Boon 2008), where culture was done routinely only for those who were positive on the screening test. A difficulty in assessing these studies is knowing exactly which diagnostic procedures were applied to the passively detected cases. Unfortunately these data were not available for most studies.

The degree of smear positivity among smear-positive cases is probably a more accurate indicator of severity. In three studies that included these data – from Cambodia, India and South Africa (den Boon 2008, Shetty 2008, Eang 2012) – the degree of smear positivity (that is, the proportion with a smear grading of 3+) was lower in screened cases. All three studies reporting radiographic grading found less extensive disease among screened cases (Ross 1977, Wang 2000, LeBue 2004). However, in none of the studies were all cases bacteriologically confirmed, and people with less severe abnormalities identified by chest radiography without independent confirmation of TB may be false positives. The possibility of length–time bias cannot be excluded.

In one study in India (Santha 2003) the proportion who had a self-reported delay of less than 3 months from the onset of symptoms until diagnosis was half among patients when compared with the proportion among passively detected cases. A study of screening among homeless people in the United Kingdom reported an average delay that was three times longer among those detected passively (Story 2012). In a Brazilian trial, at the community level there was little difference in the reported delay between intervention and control groups (Miller 2010). A cross-sectional study from Ethiopia (Shargie 2006a) found that 54% of those who had been screened had a delay of longer than 90 days compared with 58% of those who had not been screened. A community-based randomized controlled trial from Ethiopia found that the proportion of participants with a delay of longer than 90 days was 22% lower in the intervention communities (41% versus 63%). It is possible that recall bias and bias caused by different perceptions and interpretations of symptoms played a part in these studies. Such biases limit the overall quality of studies on self-reported delay. A randomized controlled trial of household screening in infants found that the time from birth to diagnosis was on average 3.4 months shorter in the screening arm (Moyo 2012).

A study from the former Czechoslovakia in the 1960s showed that 79% of people with smear-positive TB had developed the disease within 36 month of a previously normal chest X-ray. This indicated that the screening interval of 2–3 years for mass screening was too long to significantly reduce the delay in diagnosis and severity at diagnosis, at least in the context of a health-care system that ensures adequate access to high-quality health services for people seeking care for symptoms of TB (Meijer 1971). However, the proportion that developed smear-positive disease within 1 year was 17%, suggesting that an interval of 1 year or less would identify the majority of smear-positive cases earlier than passive case-finding. A 2011 study conducted among miners in South Africa (Churchyard 2011) compared 6-monthly chest X-ray screening with 12-monthly chest X-rays. TB cases detected in the 6-monthly screening arm had less extensive disease at diagnosis as judged by radiology. TB-specific mortality was lower at 2 months' follow up compared with TB cases detected in the 12-monthly screening arm; however, the mortality reduction after 12 months was not statistically significant.

Note: *Full references for the studies cited are available in the supporting material on the Internet.*

Question 3. *Is there a difference in TB treatment outcomes among cases found by screening and those found through routine passive case-finding?*

There is evidence is of very low quality that treatment outcomes among people identified through screening are similar to outcomes among those identified through passive case-finding. Details are provided in *Box 3*.

Box 3. Detailed findings for question 3: Is there a difference in TB treatment outcomes among cases found by screening and those found through routine passive case-finding?

Six studies – one in Cambodia, one in India, two in Nepal, one in South Africa and one in Zambia (Cassals 1982 , Harper 1996, Santha 2003, den Boon 2008, Ayles 2012, Eang 2012) – presented comparable data on treatment success rates for cases found through screening and those found passively. All six studies looked at community screening. The outcomes (treatment success, cure, default, failure, death) for cases found through screening and passive case-finding within each study were similar; the pooled treatment success rate ratio was 1.0 (95% confidence interval, 0.98–1.02) with low heterogeneity (I^2, 0%). In all six studies, the patients came from the same communities. However, there were many differences among the cases found through screening and those found through passive case-finding, including a tendency for cases identified through screening to have less severe disease (which would tend to give lower mortality rates but possibly higher default rates) and to be older (which would tend to give worse outcomes). The studies did not control for such baseline differences. The lack of difference in treatment outcomes is therefore difficult to interpret.

One cohort study (Churchyard 2000) assessing risk factors for case fatality in HIV-negative and HIV-positive miners with TB, found that the adjusted relative risk of death (controlling for HIV status, sputum-smear status, treatment category, age, extent of disease, silicosis and drug resistance) was 82% lower for people identified through a routine screening programme that used chest radiography compared with people identified through passive case-finding. A length–time bias and residual confounding is possible. The reduction in TB-specific mortality was much larger in the HIV-negative individuals than in the HIV-positive individuals (in whom it was not statistically significant).

The most appropriate design for assessing the impact of screening on treatment outcomes would be a controlled trial comparing treatment outcomes in a setting or a special risk group where screening is introduced to a control setting or group without screening. No such study was identified.

There are few studies comparing initial defaults (that is, people who have been diagnosed with TB but did not start treatment) between those who were detected through screening and those identified by passive case-finding. Studies conducted subsequently to the Indian study (Santha 2003) reported initial default rates for screened and passively identified cases (Gopi 2005, Balasubramanian 2004). Initial defaults were higher in screened cases (29% in 1999–2001 and 24% in 2001–2002) than in passively identified cases (14% and 15%, respectively). However, there were no deaths among the 57 people who initially defaulted after being screened, but there were 23 (19%) deaths among those who had been passively identified. The reasons given by the 57 who defaulted after having been actively identified included an unwillingness to start treatment, feeling that their symptoms were too mild to warrant treatment, they were too sick, and work-related problems (Gopi 2005). Nine additional studies (Cassels 1982, Manalo 1990, Santha 2003, Harries 2004, den Boon 2008, Corbett 2009, Eang 2012, Kranzer 2012, Okada 2012,) reported initial defaults only among screened cases; the proportions ranged from 4% to 26%. The weighted mean proportion of initial defaults in screened cases across all 10 studies was 13%, and the median was 9%. For all settings except India, initial defaults in passively identified cases were not reported, but they may be high, and such patients have poor outcomes (Hoa 2010; Ministry of Health, Cambodia, 2002; Ayles 2009; Shapiro 2012; Getahun 2011; Morrison 2008; Fox 2012).

Morbidity outcomes other than conventional TB treatment outcomes measured through cohort analyses were also considered, including relapse, acquired drug resistance, chronic sequelae, and the number of quality adjusted life-years lost. However, these data were not reported in any study.

Note: *Full references for the studies cited are available in the supporting material on the Internet.*

Question 4. *Does screening have economic and social consequences for the person with disease and his or her family?*

No studies identified either positive or negative economic or social consequences of screening.

Question 5. *Among people in TB-affected communities, does the addition of TB screening to passive case-finding affect TB epidemiology?*

The evidence is of moderate quality that implementing a screening approach that has low sensitivity does not affect TB epidemiology. The evidence ranges from very low quality to low quality that more intensive screening can reduce the burden of TB in the screened population. Details are provided in *Box 4*.

Box 4. **Detailed findings for question 5: Among people in TB-affected communities, does the addition of TB screening to passive case-finding affect TB epidemiology?**

Five studies provided evidence for the effect of TB screening on the burden of TB in the general population.

Of these studies, two were randomized controlled trials comparing screening with no screening. The first was the Zambia-South Africa TB and AIDS Reduction programme study (ZAMSTAR), which was conducted in communities in Zambia and South Africa. ZAMSTAR had a 2 x 2 factorial design comparing (1) a community-outreach intervention that included health-information campaigns and decentralized and easy-access sputum collection; (2) a household intervention that included repeated rounds of investigations of contacts of people with TB, HIV counselling and testing, isoniazid preventive treatment and general health information; (3) the interventions described in (1) and (2); or (4) no intervention (Ayles 2012). The outcomes that were assessed included the prevalence of TB as determined by surveys and the incidence of infection with *Mycobacterium tuberculosis*, which was assessed by evaluating tuberculin conversion in children. The community intervention had no impact on the prevalence of TB or the incidence of TB infection. The household intervention (which reached 6% of individuals in the community) was associated with a reduction in the burden of TB in the community: there was a 22% lower prevalence of active TB and a 55% lower incidence of TB infection. However, the reductions were not statistically significant. The second trial took place in Brazil: four matched pairs of communities were randomized to receive intensive household screening of contacts (including tuberculin skin testing and isoniazid prophylaxis) (Cavalcante 2010), while the control communities received the standard DOTS package for TB care. Outcomes were assessed using TB registration data, and the denominator was taken from the national census. Overall, TB notifications decreased by 10% in the intervention communities and increased by 5% in the control communities, but information on long-term trends in incidence were not presented.

A community-based randomized trial in Zimbabwe (known as DETECTB) used two different case-finding interventions (mobile vans or door-to-door visits) (Corbett 2010). There was no control group without an intervention, so TB prevalence in the communities before and after the intervention was assessed by conducting prevalence surveys. Prevalence was reduced by 40% over 3 years in both arms of the trial. The reduction was similar in areas covered by the different interventions, although the cumulative yield of cases during the intervention was higher in the group covered by the mobile van. The population of the area increased by 10% during the study period (January 2006 to November 2008), which may have influenced the prevalence of TB.

Two studies assessed secular trends in screened populations. A follow-up study was conducted in Cambodia 2 years after a national survey of TB prevalence to capture incident cases of TB in community clusters that had been screened for TB as part of the national survey (Okada 2012). The standardized notification ratio for TB was 62% lower in the communities that had been screened than what would have been expected had the communities followed national trends. A study in the United States evaluated a programme of mandatory screening plus mandatory prophylaxis and treatment when indicated for those wanting to use homeless shelters (Rendlemann 1999). Trends in tuberculosis in the whole district fell by almost 90% over 10 years. The statewide incidence of TB was much lower, but areas other than the intervention area showed no such fall. The study did not assess the effect of screening alone, and the population of the district changed during the study period as a result of gentrification, so this may have contributed to some of the fall.

Overall, the evidence remains weak for the impact of screening on TB epidemiology in the community. Only a few studies have been published, and these assess just a few of the many possible screening approaches in only a limited number of epidemiological contexts. Most studies have important methodological limitations. Two studies (Cavalcante 2010, Ayles 2012) found a decline in TB in the community associated with the screening of TB contacts, but screening for active TB was a only part of a larger intervention package. Two studies (Corbett 2010, Okada 2012) found a decline in TB prevalence and notification rates associated with community screening. Corbett 2010 had no control arm without screening, and in Cambodia, Okada 2012 compared notification in screened communities only with the national average. The fifth study (Rendlemann 1999) found a rapidly declining secular trend in TB notification associated with the introduction of screening in homeless shelters, but the study had no formal control areas.

Note: *Full references for the studies cited are available in the supporting material on the Internet.*

5.2 Review 2: systematic review of the sensitivity and specificity of different screening tools and algorithms

The full review can be found in the supporting material available at www.who.int/tb/tbscreening.

Screening in adults

The pooled sensitivity and specificity of screening tests, using culture-confirmed pulmonary TB as the gold standard, are summarized in *Table 2*. GRADE tables assessing the quality of the evidence are provided in *Annex II*.

Table 2. **Pooled sensitivity and specificity of different screening tools for pulmonary tuberculosis (TB), using culture-confirmed pulmonary TB as the gold standard**

Screening tool	Pooled sensitivity % (95% confidence interval)	Pooled specificity % (95% confidence interval
Chest radiography		
Any abnormality compatible with TB (active or inactive)	98 (95–100)	75 (72–79)
Abnormalities suggestive of active TB	87 (79–95)	89 (87–92)
After positive screening for symptoms[a]	90 (81–96)	56 (54–58)
Symptom screening		
Prolonged cough (lasting >2–3 weeks)	35 (24–46)	95 (93–97)
Any cough	57 (40–74)	80 (69–90)
Any TB symptom (settings with low prevalence of HIV)	70 (58–82)	61 (35–87)
Any TB symptom (settings with high prevalence of HIV)	84 (76–93)	74 (53–95)
Any TB symptom (settings with low prevalence or high prevalence of HIV)	77 (68–86)	68 (50–85)

[a] Results from only one study, data for any abnormality on chest radiography.

The yield of different screening and diagnostic algorithms was estimated using the point estimates for sensitivity and specificity for different screening tools (*Table 2*) and the pooled point estimates from systematic reviews of the sensitivity and specificity of the Xpert MTB/RIF[49] test and sputum-smear microscopy [50,51] using culture-confirmed pulmonary TB as the gold standard (*Table 3*). The sensitivity and specificity of clinical diagnosis (that is, clinical evaluation plus chest radiography of patients with smear-negative TB) were taken from an economic evaluation by Vassall and colleagues[52] that used findings from a demonstration study of the Xpert MTB/RIF test in three countries.

Table 3. **Sensitivity and specificity of different diagnostic tests from systematic reviews, using culture-confirmed pulmonary tuberculosis (TB) as the gold standard**

Diagnostic test	Sensitivity % (95% confidence interval)	Specificity % (95% confidence interval)
Liquid culture (gold standard)	100	100
Conventional sputum-smear microscopy[50,51]	61 (31–89)	98 (93–100)
Xpert MTB/RIF[49]	92 (70–100)	99 (91–100)
Clinical diagnosis[52] [a]	24 (10–51)	94 (79–97)

[a] Clinical evaluation plus chest radiography after negative sputum-smear microscopy or Xpert MTB/RIF. Part of the study population was declared TB-negative based on having a good response to broad spectrum antibiotics, which were given before chest radiography was done. Using chest radiography as a diagnostic test for smear-negative TB (rather than an algorithm that includes broad spectrum antibiotics, chest radiography and repeat smears) would have a higher sensitivity but a lower specificity compared with the estimates in the table.

Table 4. Modelled yield of different algorithms when screening 100 000 persons in a population with a 1% prevalence of culture positive pulmonary TB (1 000 cases). (It is assumed that the final diagnosis uses results from sputum-smear microscopy or the Xpert MTB/RIF test, and there is no further diagnostic evaluation)[a]

Screening	Final diagnostic test	Outcome of screening[a]						Outcome of diagnosis in persons with positive screening[a]				
		TN	FN	NPV[b] (%)	Screened positive[c]	TP	Detected of true cases (%)	FP	PPV[d] (%)	TN[e] (n)	FN[f]	NPV[g] (%)
Cough lasting >2 weeks	SSM	93 753	649	99.3	5 598	214	21	105	67.1	5 142	137	97.4
	Xpert	93 753	649	99.3	5 598	324	32	52	86.0	5 195	27	99.5
1st screen: cough >2 weeks 2nd screen: (if 1st screen positive): chest radiography	SSM	96 691	684	99.3	2 625	193	19	46	80.7	2 263	123	94.8
	Xpert	96 691	684	99.3	2 625	291	29	23	92.7	2 286	25	98.9
Any TB symptom	SSM	67 023	230	99.7	32 747	470	47	640	42.3	31 337	300	99.
	Xpert	67 023	230	99.7	32 747	710	71	320	68.9	31 657	60	99.8
1st screen: any TB symptom 2nd screen (if 1st screen positive): chest radiography	SSM	84 930	307	99.6	14 763	423	42	281	60.0	13 788	270	98.
	Xpert	84 930	307	99.6	14 763	639	64	141	82.0	13 929	54	99.6
Chest radiography: abnormality suggestive of active TB	SSM	88 506	132	99.9	11 362	529	53	210	71.6	10 284	339	96.
	Xpert	88 506	132	99.9	11 362	800	80	105	88.4	10 389	68	99.
Chest radiography: any abnormality compatible with TB	SSM	74 646	22	100.0	25 332	597	60	487	55.1	23 867	381	98.
	Xpert	74 646	22	100.0	25 332	902	90	244	78.7	24 110	76	99.

TN, true negative; FN, false negative; NPV, negative predictive value; TP, true positive; FP, false positive; PPV, positive predictive value; SSM, sputum-smear microscopy; Xpert, Xpert MTB/RIF test.
[a] Values are numbers unless otherwise indicated.
[b] The negative predictive value for screening is the likelihood that someone whose screening test is negative does not have TB.
[c] This is the number of people whose screening test would be positive, which equals the number of people who should have the diagnostic test
[d] The positive predictive value is the likelihood that a person with a final diagnosis of TB has true culture-positive TB.
[e] The number of true negatives among people screened positive is the number of people correctly diagnosed as not having TB among those whose screening tests is positive and who has a diagnostic test.
[f] The number of false negatives among people whose screening is positive is the number of people falsely diagnosed as not having TB among those whose screening tests is positive and who has a diagnostic test.
[g] The negative predictive value for diagnosis among people whose screening was positive is the likelihood that a person whose screening test is positive and who is not diagnosed with TB does not have culture-positive TB.

The modelled yields of different algorithms when screening 100 000 persons in a population with a 1% prevalence of TB are shown in *Table 4*. These scenarios assume that the final diagnosis uses results from sputum-smear microscopy or the Xpert MTB/RIF test, and that there is no further diagnostic evaluation. (The modelled yields of the same scenarios, and scenarios including further diagnostic evaluation of those who have negative results on their diagnostic test, at different prevalence levels – 0.5%, 1% and 2% – are shown in the supporting material available at www.who.int/tb/tbscreening. This material also includes the modelled number of tests required per each true case detected.)

Screening in children
Only two studies fulfilled the inclusion criteria for the systematic review.

One study assessed symptom screening in children aged younger than 5 years who were contacts of someone with TB.[53] The presence of cough, fever, weight loss or fatigue had a sensitivity of 76% and specificity of 77%, with a positive predictive value of 33% and a negative predictive value of 96%; the study population had a TB prevalence of 13%. Among the eight children whose screening test was negative and who were diagnosed with active TB in the study, all had only hilar adenopathy identified by chest radiography; this was interpreted as probable transient hilar adenopathy occurring after infection rather than as active TB disease. Although these children were treated for active TB in the study, the authors concluded that it would have been safe to treat such children for latent TB instead.

One study[54] assessed a screening algorithm for HIV-positive children. The presence of cough lasting longer than 2 weeks, fever or failure to thrive had a sensitivity 95% and a specificity 59%. The absence of these symptoms had a negative predictive value of 99%.

No other studies assessing screening algorithms for use in children were identified, although several studies have assessed the sensitivity and specificity of different diagnostic approaches in populations of children who were already suspected of having TB. These studies were not included in the review.

5.3 Review 3: systematic review of the number needed to screen in different risk groups

This review included 727 studies. *Table 5* summarizes the weighted average number needed to screen (NNS) to find one case of TB in different risk groups in different epidemiological situations. (The full review, including median and interquartile ranges for NNS can be found in the supporting material available at www.who.int/tb/tbscreening.)

Table 5. **Weighted mean and range number needed to screen (NNS) to find one case of tuberculosis (TB) in selected risk categories. All screening approaches are aggregated within each risk group**

Population screened (No. of studies)	Low incidence (<30/100,000)	Moderate incidence (30-100/100,000)	Medium incidence (100-300/100,000)	High incidence (>300/100,000)
General population (98)	3922 (137–30865)[a]	669 (15–5594)	603 (25–4286)	100 (16–6355)
Infants in vaccine trial (3)	NS	NS	140 (7–343)	NS
Immigrants (26)	235 (3–1262)[a]	NS	1206 (198–6250)	NS
Refugees (38)	108 (6–1630)[a]		120 (57–291)	
Military (6)	1159 (134–492)[a]	NS	1280 (73–1440)	NS
Health-care workers (16)	1613 (30–5550)[a]		506 (25–842)[a]	NS
Miners (8)	48 (–)[b]	154 (–)[b]	NS	36 (21–93)
Other occupations (14)	1565 (47–5235)[a]	NS	109 (4–778)	NS
Homeless people (18)	133 (22–1778)	NS	NS	NS
Prisoners (44)	1180 (4–2945)[a]	155 (19–191)	110 (7–2762)	
General inpatients (4)	NS	NS	795 (6–3364)	
General outpatients (14)	758 (42–30 000)		269 (19–806)	
Nursing homes (7)	120 (68–137)[a]		NS	7 (–)[b]
Psychiatric facilities (3)	1049 (32–1275)		111 (–)[b]	NS
Pregnant women (9)	536 (88–3843)[a]	NS	36 (25–143)	
People with diabetes (6)	NS	2223 (–)[b]	35 (17–54)	
Drug users (8)	158 (108–252)[a]	5 (–)[b]	20 (8–20)	NS
VCTC (5)	NS		37 (8–120)	
People living with HIV (74)	30 (8–391)[a]	61 (5–316)	13 (2–120)[a]	10 (3–64)
Other clinical groups (6)	290 (10–2846)[a]	NS	4 (–)[b]	NS
Gynaecology clinics (5)	18 (–)[b]	NS	13 (5–38)	
Household contacts (89)	54 (5–430)[a]	40 (7–355)[a]	25 (3–568)[a]	17 (2–129)
Community contacts (78)	104 (3–4200)[a]	85 (6–137)	NS	
Health-care contacts (17)	276 (7–223)[a]	25 (–)[b]	NS	NS

NS, no study for risk group in the incidence category; VCTC, voluntary counselling and testing for HIV
[a] The true upper range of the NNS was not defined because one or several studies found no cases of TB. The highest definable NNS is reported here as the upper limit of the range.
[b] In cases in which there was only one study, no range is given.

5.4 Review 4: systematic review of the acceptability of screening

A total of 468 studies were included in the systematic review, and 218 (47%) of these evaluated voluntary screening and contained detailed information on the proportion of eligible individuals who accepted screening. (The full review can be found in the supporting material available at www.who.int/tb/tbscreening.)

Table 6 shows the average, range and median proportion of eligible persons who consented to undergo TB screening. The only groups in which consent rates were below 80% were indigenous populations, persons being tested for HIV, people attending health centres, men who have sex with men and health-care workers, but most median rates were still above 80%. *Table 7* shows the consent rates for contact investigation.

The consent rate is an indirect indicator of the acceptability of testing. Few studies assessed acceptability from the perspective of people offered screening and then analysed the factors that determined acceptability. A summary of a qualitative assessment of the evidence is presented in *Box 5*.

Table 6. **Proportion of persons accepting tuberculosis (TB) screening in 218 studies, by risk group[a]**

Risk group	Mean	Weighted mean	No.of studies	Minimum	Maximum	Median
Members of the military[b]	96	99	2	93	100	96
Farm and factory workers[b]	97	97	3	95	98	98
Homeless people[b]	66	96	5	41	97	75
People with mental illness	94	95	2	93	95	94
People with diabetes	96	94	2	94	98	96
Pregnant women	85	94	6	68	96	90
People with drug dependencies[b]	84	93	3	69	94	89
Urban residents of poor areas	87	91	11	59	99	88
Sex workers	86	84	2	84	88	88
Children younger than 5 years	87	87	2	84	91	86
Transport workers[b]	85	86	3	73	98	84
Migrants	77	85	8	55	96	81
HIV-positive PMTCT [b,c]	79	81	3	68	96	88
Adolescents	72	80	3	58	96	79
Transgender people[b]	77	79	2	77	91	84
People living with HIV	82	78	17	52	99	83
Refugees or internally displaced	51	72	2	23	79	51
Elderly people living in institutions[b]	83	72	2	72	95	83
Prisoners	71	72	16	18	98	86
Miners	81	70	6	66	93	84
Indigenous people	82	69	9	40	97	89
People being tested for HIV	73	69	5	41	97	85
Men who have sex with men (MSM)	76	61	2	64	91	76
Attendees at health centres	59	68	3	52	67	57
Health-care workers[b]	78	59	5	56	91	80
Refugees	41	54	2	23	74	41

[a] Values are percentages unless otherwise indicated.
[b] In these cases, consent also included consent to tuberculin skin testing.
[c] Pregnant HIV-positive women in programmes for preventing mother-to-child transmission

Table 7. **Acceptability of contact investigation for tuberculosis by type**[a]

Type of contact tracing	No. of studies	Mean	Minimum	Maximum	Median
Household	24	80	39	99	85
Community	27	88	57	100	91
In health-care settings	4	59	43	73	60
Other	3	87	83	95	84

[a] Values are percentages unless otherwise indicated.

Box 5. **Summary of a qualitative assessment of evidence on the acceptability of screening for TB**

A qualitative assessment of the evidence on the acceptability of screening for TB suggested that acceptability is influenced by:
- the screening test used, particularly whether it is invasive or noninvasive;
- the time required for the test and follow-up visit;
- the perceived negative consequences of screening (such as, legal, social, political and economic consequences);
- the incentives offered;
- the quality of the interaction with the person doing the screening;
- the number of times screening is repeated.

Specifically:
- simple TB screening (that is, a one-step point–of-care process) is more acceptable to almost all groups studied than is referral for testing or testing that involves multiple visits;
- simple TB screening is more acceptable than more complex, invasive screening that involves blood draws, gastric aspiration or hospital admission;
- acceptability declines over time when screening is offered multiple times; acceptability may be a function of periodicity, so the intervals between screening tests should balance the health benefits against the increasing risk of refusal;
- including HIV testing in the TB screening algorithm (or a person's fear that HIV testing will be included) may deter some risk groups (for example, health-care workers), however inclusion of HIV testing in TB screening was not found to increase refusal in community-based TB screening.
- TB screening and treatment may be low priorities for groups facing housing insecurity, nutritional insecurity, addiction, the threat of violence or deportation;
- screening is more acceptable to hard-to-reach street populations if the benefits are immediate and tangible, as they are with the use of incentives and enablers.

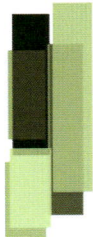

6. Assessing TB screening against generic criteria for screening

Table 8 lists generally agreed criteria for determining when disease screening is appropriate, and evaluates screening for active TB against those criteria.

Screening for disease is appropriate only if it can efficiently detect disease at an early stage, and if early treatment has significantly better outcomes than later treatment.[55,56] The outcomes of interest both occur on the individual level and, in the case of communicable diseases, on the community level, through the impact that screening has on transmission. Screening is particularly appropriate for conditions that are nonsymptomatic or have only vague symptoms during the early stages that are unlikely to be recognized by the person with the disease. While screening can detect many diseases early and with high precision, the critical question is whether the disease can be detected and treated early enough, and at a reasonable cost, to significantly change the outcomes of disease.

In theory, screening for active TB can improve tertiary prevention by enabling treatment to be initiated earlier, thus reducing the risk of poor treatment outcomes, the risk of long-term sequelae and the adverse socioeconomic consequences of TB. If screening for active TB reduces the delay in diagnosis, for which there is some evidence,[57] it is plausible that it should enable treatment to be started earlier and thereby reduce the risk of poor outcomes, especially in groups with a high baseline risk of poor treatment outcomes. However, there is no direct evidence that screening in these and other groups can reduce the risk of adverse outcomes[58] (see Section 5.1 and *Annex 1* in this document, and the supporting material available at www.who.int/tb/tbscreening). Thus, while diagnosing and treating a person with previously undetected TB disease significantly benefits both the individual and society when compared with not providing treatment, it is still uncertain whether screening for active TB followed by delivering appropriate treatment leads to better health outcomes than passive case-finding followed by appropriate treatment.

Screening may also improve primary prevention by reducing the transmission of TB. However, whether this potential benefit occurs is uncertain, even in theory, owing to some critical gaps in our understanding of the natural history of TB, including the relationship between the progression of TB symptoms or signs and TB transmission. The exact timing of transmission events and the proportion of these that would be prevented by detecting cases early through systematic screening is not fully understood, and the timing may differ among groups and lineages of *Mycobacterium tuberculosis*. If smear-positive disease develops quickly in predisposed individuals alongside rapidly progressive TB symptoms, while patients with smear-negative disease tend to progress slowly over long periods of time, then in the presence of readily accessible health services for those who feel ill, screening would have relatively little impact on transmission, regardless of the screening interval. At the other extreme, if smear-positivity develops early on in the course of TB disease despite a prolonged subclinical stage, and most smear-negative TB patients convert to being smear-positive over time, then screening even at moderate-to-long intervals will prevent substantial amounts of smear-positive time, thereby preventing secondary infections. Ultimately, the proof that screening has an impact on transmission needs to be established through randomized trials that compare screening with alternative interventions. However, the evidence remains weak since only a few controlled trials have been conducted, they have used a variety of approaches, are of variable quality and have had mixed findings[58] (see Section 5.1 and *Annex 1* in this document, and in the supporting material available at www.who.int/tb/tbscreening).

When there is little empirical evidence, mathematical modelling can help create scenarios to assess the possible impacts, but these scenarios require verification through clinical trials. Mathematical modelling suggests that screening for active TB may help reduce transmission and incidence,[58,59] and thereby reduce the future costs of TB care,[60] under certain conditions. Modelling also suggests that screening in transmission hot spots may be particularly efficient in reducing transmission both within and outside hot spots – for example, in poor urban areas[61] and prisons.[62] However, without reliable parameters for the natural course of TB or estimates from empirical studies of the impact of screening on transmission, such models should be interpreted with caution.

Table 8. **Assessing the appropriateness of screening for active tuberculosis (TB) against WHO's generic criteria for disease screening**

Wilson and Jungner's criteria for determining whether disease screening is appropriate*	Screening for TB	
	Criteria fulfilled?	Comment
1. Condition is an important health problem for the individual and community	Yes	In settings with a high burden of TB the criteria is fulfilled because of the health and economic burdens of TB. In low-burden countries each case of TB is a potential outbreak that must be contained.
2. There is accepted treatment for patients with the disease	Yes	Untreated TB is associated with a high case-fatality rate, about 70% for smear-positive TB and 20% for smear-negative.[63] TB treatment can reduce the case-fatality rate to about 3% (among people who are HIV-negative).[64] Standard treatment for drug-susceptible TB usually renders an infectious individual noninfectious within 2–3 weeks. However, there is mixed evidence on the association between case-fatality and delayed diagnosis.[65] TB is associated with considerable loss of quality of life both during and after active TB disease. However, the association between a delay in diagnosis and the risk of sequelae has not been established.[66] Active TB can arise from recent infection or from latent infection. Active TB can have an early subclinical stage, during which symptoms are absent, or an early symptomatic stage, during which symptoms progress from vague and moderate to more prominent. Infectiousness correlates with the severity of signs and symptoms.[67,68] However, there is insufficient evidence on the natural rate of progression of signs and symptoms, the rate of natural recovery, the natural rate of progression of infectiousness, and the association among these parameters.
3. The natural history of the disease should be adequately understood	Conditionally	
4. There should be a latent or early symptomatic stage	Yes	
5. There should be a suitable and acceptable screening test	Yes	Screening for symptoms or screening with chest radiography, or both, are suitable[69] and acceptable[70] tools for diagnosing pulmonary TB in most risk groups and most settings.

6.Facilities for diagnosis and treatment should be available.	Conditionally	Accurate diagnostic tools for pulmonary TB, highly effective treatments, and internationally agreed standards for diagnosis and treatment are available.[71] However, there is a risk of false-positive and false-negative diagnoses with all diagnostic tools; also, the quality of diagnostic services, and the provision and accessibility of treatment, varies across settings. This criteria therefore needs to be assessed separately for different diagnostic tests and in relation to local diagnostic and treatment capacities.
7.There should be an agreed policy on whom to treat as patients	Yes	There is an internationally agreed case definition for TB, although uncertainty remains about culture-negative pulmonary TB, extrapulmonary TB and TB in children. In addition, there is no consensus on whether to define a person with positive sputum bacteriology but no symptoms and no abnormalities identified by chest radiography as having active TB.
8.Early treatment has more benefit than treatment started later	Yes	The shorter the period of infectiousness, the less transmission. It is plausible that the risk of poor outcomes, death and subsequent sequelae increases with delay, but the direct evidence on the exact relationship between delay and adverse outcome is weak (see above).
9.The cost should be economically balanced	Conditionally	Cost may be assessed in relation to the number of additional cases detected, the reduction in transmission, the reduction in suffering and death, and the social and economic impacts on individuals and society. Costs and relative cost effectiveness depend on the risk group, the screening approach, the alternative interventions and the local epidemiology of TB. Therefore, the judgement of benefits in relation to costs needs to be assessed locally and separately for different risk groups.

* Wilson JMG, Jungner G. *Principles and practice of screening for disease*. Geneva, World Health Organization, 1968.

Table 8 shows that three of the generic criteria for screening are only conditionally fulfilled by screening for active TB:

- criterion 3 – although the natural history of TB infection and disease progression is generally known, they are not adequately understood to allow definitive conclusions to be drawn;
- criterion 6 – the availability of high-quality diagnosis and treatment varies greatly in different settings. This criterion needs to be assessed locally;
- criterion 9 – the final criterion, which assesses benefits in relation to costs, depends on many factors, including the local epidemiology, the risk groups targeted, the screening approach used, and the costs and effects of alternative interventions.

There are several scenarios under which TB screening potentially could fulfil all of the generic criteria for screening, notably in areas where the burden is high and where the baseline delay until diagnosis and treatment is long and associated with severe adverse outcomes for individuals or with a high rate of transmission, or both. However, there are also situations in which TB screening can do more harm than good – for example, this would be the case if screening leads to only a marginal positive effect on morbidity and transmission but the cost is high and screening generates large numbers of false-positive cases. This scenario is more likely to occur in settings or populations with a low-to-moderate burden of TB in which the baseline delay until diagnosis and treatment is short. Therefore, the screening criteria need to be assessed separately for different epidemiological situations and for different risk groups.

The recommendations developed by the Guideline Development Group (see Section 8) used separate assessments for each risk group considered, and take account of different epidemiological situations.

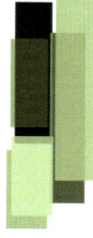

7. Key principles for screening for active TB

Principle 1: Before screening is initiated, high-quality TB diagnosis, treatment, care, management and support for patients should be in place, and there should be the capacity to scale these up further to match the anticipated rise in case detection that may occur as a result of screening. In addition, a baseline analysis should be completed in order to demonstrate that the potential benefits of screening clearly outweigh the risks of doing harm, and that the required investments in screening are reasonable in relation to the expected benefits.

The following key conditions should be met before screening is initiated.

- High-quality TB diagnosis, treatment, management and support for patients should be in place. The critical conditions that must be met include ensuring that good-quality diagnostic services are available as well as a regular supply of anti-TB medicines, that there are sufficient mechanisms to provide support for patients, and that there is a low rate of initial default (that is, people who are diagnosed with TB but who do not begin treatment). There must be adequate capacity for culture and drug-susceptibility testing. There must be capacity for the programmatic management of drug-resistant TB, at least in settings with a moderate-to-high prevalence of drug-resistant TB. There must be capacity to scale up services while ensuring that barriers to accessing treatment are minimized for those who are identified through screening. There must be adequate financial resources and human resources. There must be the capacity to tailor treatment programmes to the specific needs of the screened population. If necessary, additional resources should be made available but making resources available for screening should not have an adverse impact on other key functions of the health-care system.

- Baseline epidemiological analyses and health-system situation analyses must be done before screening is implemented. Analyses of existing legal and human rights frameworks must also be completed. The potential benefits and harms of screening must be analysed to determine whether the benefits of screening are likely to outweigh the risks of doing harm. An assessment must be made to determine whether the required investments are reasonable in relation to the expected benefits and when compared with alternative interventions. Specifically, opportunities and barriers to improving passive case-finding approaches should be analysed to determine whether screening is an important and cost-effective complement.

Principle 2: Indiscriminate mass screening should be avoided. The prioritization of risk groups for screening should be based on assessments made for each risk group of the potential benefits and harms, the feasibility of the initiative, the acceptability of the approach, the number needed to screen, and the cost effectiveness of screening.

Section 8 presents the recommendations made by the Guideline Development Group on which risk groups should be considered for screening. Several of the recommendations are conditional, implying that prioritization is needed; this prioritization must be based on the epidemiological situation, the health-system context and the availability of resources.

Prioritization may vary depending on which stakeholder is responsible for the screening initiative. For example, a national TB programme under the auspice of a ministry of health may have other mandates, priorities and resources than health services that fall under a ministry of justice, ministry of labour, immigration authorities, nongovernmental organizations, private health-care providers or employers.

When prioritizing which groups to screen, the following factors should be considered for each risk group.

- **Potential benefits for the individual:** These benefits include the health, social and economic benefits of early diagnosis and treatment of TB. In principle, the potential benefits are greater for persons who have a high risk of delaying diagnosis because there are barriers to health care, or they have a high risk of poor treatment outcome when diagnosis is delayed –for example, because their immune system is compromised.

- **Potential risks for the individual:** These risks are associated with the process of screening and diagnosis and include the time, inconvenience and cost of screening, as well as the result of screening. Harms from the results of screening include the unintended negative effects of being correctly diagnosed (which may cause stigma or discrimination) and harm caused by a false-positive diagnosis or a false-negative diagnosis.

- **Potential impact on transmission within and beyond the risk group:** The potential of screening to have an impact on transmission is theoretically highest in congregate settings where there is a high rate of transmission and where there is also substantial in-migration and out-migration. In principle, the larger the risk group that is screened, the larger the potential impact on transmission in the community. However, when the TB burden is highly concentrated in a few high-risk groups, the largest impact on overall transmission may come from screening highly selected groups, and these may be small in size.

- **Feasibility and acceptability of identifying, reaching and screening people in the risk group, and having them start and complete treatment**: It is generally more feasible to conduct screening in well defined risk groups that are possible to reach in a specific location – for example, among clinical risk groups identified within health facilities, among people who are in institutions (such as prisons), and in high-risk workplaces (such as mines).

- **The number needed to screen to detect a case of TB, and the related estimated cost per each true case detected:** The number needed to screen declines as the prevalence of undetected TB increases; therefore, the number is lowest in risk groups with the highest burden of undetected TB. However, the number needed to screen also depends on the accuracy of the screening and the diagnostic algorithm used.

- **Cost effectiveness, and cost benefit:** Cost effectiveness can be estimated in relation to the number of additional true TB cases detected, the reduction in morbidity, the reduced time that a person remains infectious, and the reductions in transmission, incidence and mortality. Cost benefit can be estimated in terms of future costs saved for the individual, the health sector or society, or all of these. The total cost depends on the number needed to screen, the algorithm used for screening and diagnosis, the method used to reach people for screening, and the direct and indirect costs incurred for the screened individuals.

Principle 3: The choice of algorithm for screening and diagnosis should be based on an assessment of the accuracy of the algorithm for each risk group considered, as well as the availability, feasibility and cost of the tests.

The likelihood of a correct diagnosis (a true positive or true negative) and the risk of an incorrect diagnosis (a false positive or false negative) depend on:
- the sensitivity and specificity of the screening tool;
- the sensitivity and specificity of the diagnostic tool;
- the prevalence of undetected TB in the screened population.

The expected yield of the algorithm, the predictive values, and modelled number of tests required to detect each true case of TB for different algorithms at different levels of TB prevalence are provided in Section 5.2, and *Annex III*.

The algorithms assume that sputum-smear microscopy or the Xpert MTB/RIF test (or any rapid test recommended by WHO in the future that has the same or better accuracy) is used as a final diagnostic test, or that further clinical diagnosis is considered for those with a negative result on the diagnostic test. To improve the positive predictive value of the final diagnosis, a repeat test or culture (and drug-susceptibility testing) may be considered for people with a positive diagnostic test. These options are not included in the modelled output of different algorithms.

The consequences of true and false diagnostic outcomes should be considered separately for each risk group considered (see Section 7.2).

The diagnostic test should include drug-susceptibility testing for people at high risk of drug-resistant TB. When a diagnostic test with integrated drug-susceptibility testing (such as the Xpert MTB/RIF) is used in an algorithm, there should be capacity for full drug-susceptibility testing as well as programmatic management of drug-resistant TB.

The availability of screening tests and diagnostic tests, as well as the costs, human-resource requirements and feasibility of introducing new tests should be considered. In principle, the diagnostic tool used in algorithms for screening and diagnosis should be the same as the diagnostic tools used for general TB diagnosis. New, more sensitive and more specific tests should be introduced first in the general diagnostic services before being used as part of a screening strategy, or they should be introduced in parallel, unless the tests are particularly suitable for screening .

Principle 4: TB screening should follow established ethical principles for screening for infectious diseases, observe human rights, and be designed to minimize the risk of discomfort, pain, stigma and discrimination.

The following key ethical principles should be followed.

- **Informed consent:** Participants should always be informed about the procedure; the implications of the test results, including the potential benefits and harms of screening; and the potential harms of not being screened. This should be done in language that has been adapted to and is suitable for the participants to ensure that they understand the information. In cases where the public-health benefits of screening justify opt-out screening, this may be used as the default option, for reasons of efficiency and for reasons of public-health ethics, but participants should have the right to decline. In special circumstances, screening may be mandatory – for example, in cases where there is a clear risk to household contacts, or as a condition of employment. Once the test is done, the screening programme has an ethical obligation to give feedback about the test results and provide high-quality treatment for any disease detected. If possible, aggregated information should be provided to the screened population. Proper management or referral for conditions other than TB that may be detected during screening should be ensured, and identified risk factors (including those that are clinical, behavioural, social or economic) should be addressed.

- **Privacy and confidentiality:** The privacy and confidentiality of screening-related information should be ensured. Confidentiality may be breached ethically and legally only for purposes of case-based surveillance.

Confidentiality may be compromised when close contacts are informed that they may have been exposed to a disease. Breaches of confidentiality should be restricted to the minimum necessary for public-health purposes.

- **Protecting vulnerable populations:** The risk of discrimination and stigmatization should be carefully assessed prior to initiating screening. Depending on the identified risks for different target groups, measures should be adapted to minimize consequences. In particular, the legal status of migrants, both with regards to access to health services and risks of expatriation in case of TB diagnosis, need to be fully considered when designing the screening approach. Similarly, when screening is conducted among specific occupational groups the legal protection of workers' rights to care and to maintain employment should be considered.

As for other health interventions, people approached for TB screening should be involved in designing screening programmes.

Principle 5: The TB screening approach should be developed and implemented in a way that optimizes synergies with the delivery of other health services and social services.

TB screening should be appropriately coordinated and integrated with other health-care services and health-promotion activities. Combining screening for other conditions or risk factors with TB screening should be considered; and mechanisms for referring and managing patients should be established from the outset. This will help optimize the use of resources. It may also increase the relevance and attractiveness of the screening activity to the target population, since it may improve access to several health-promotion and health-care interventions.

As part of the preparation for implementing screening, the structure of relevant clinical services should be assessed with the aim of exploring possibilities for collaboration across different disciplines that need to be involved in TB screening for specific risk groups, such as HIV clinics, diabetes clinics, antenatal clinics, substance abuse clinics, and general outpatient departments. Reciprocal screening should be considered – for example, people with TB should be screened for HIV and diabetes.

Screening platforms and other outreach activities may also be suitable for TB screening, such as strategies used for screening for noncommunicable diseases, childhood malnutrition, malaria or HIV. Similarly, health services and social services that target special populations – such as prisoners, homeless people, refugees, people living in remote areas or those living in slums – may be suitable as platforms for implementing TB screening.

Potential partners in developing, implementing and evaluating screening approaches also include health services that fall under the jurisdiction of ministries other than ministries of health (such as, justice or labour) and other government authorities (such as those concerned with immigration) as well as private health-care providers, nongovernmental organizations and civil society organizations.

Principle 6: A screening strategy should be monitored and reassessed continually to inform re- prioritization of risk groups, re-adaptation of screening approaches when necessary and discontinuation of screening at an appropriate time.

A plan for monitoring and evaluation should be developed before a screening initiative is launched. Indicators, data-collection forms and routines need to be adapted to the specific objectives of screening and to local conditions.

When a national or subnational screening strategy is designed, important information gaps may be uncovered. To monitor the yield of screening in each targeted risk group, an appropriate information system needs to be developed to generate data on the number of people diagnosed with TB in relation to the number of people approached and screened. The general epidemiology of TB, the importance of different risk groups, as well as the epidemiology of TB within each group may change over time, and prioritization for TB screening will have to be adapted accordingly.

Targets should be set for the expected yield, the number needed to screen and costs in relation to benefits. General conditions for discontinuing screening and conditions specific to different risk groups should be established from the outset; these may be set in relation to the number needed to screen, the contribution of screening to overall case detection, or the cost per true case detected, or some combination of these.

See Section 10 for information on suggestions for indicators to be used for monitoring and evaluating screening.

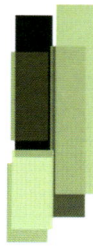

8. Recommendations on risk groups to be screened for active TB

Strong recommendations and conditional recommendations are presented separately.

Strong recommendations (Recommendations 1–3) are those for which the desirable effects of adhering to the recommendation are judged to clearly outweigh the undesirable effects; for these recommendations screening is judged to be feasible, acceptable and affordable in all settings. The Guideline Development Group placed a high value on ensuring that TB is diagnosed early in groups with a particularly high likelihood of having undetected TB and at a high risk for poor health outcomes in the absence of early diagnosis and treatment even if direct evidence of the benefits of screening were lacking. This is the rationale for making strong recommendations despite a lack of high-quality direct evidence for some risk groups.

Conditional recommendations (recommendations 4–7) are those for which the desirable effects of adhering to the recommendation probably outweigh the undesirable effects but the trade-offs, cost effectiveness, feasibility or affordability, or a combination of these, are uncertain. Reasons for uncertainty may include:
- a lack of high-quality evidence to support the recommendation;
- evidence of limited benefits from implementing the recommendation;
- high costs, or low feasibility or acceptability, or a combination of these.

The degree of uncertainty about the trade-offs between the desirable effects and undesirable effects of adhering to each of the conditional recommendations varies across settings, and depends on the epidemiological situation and the health system. Therefore, a conditional recommendation in this guideline implies that:
- the appropriateness of adhering to the recommendation needs to be assessed in each setting; and

- there is a need to prioritize screening across risk groups in each setting.

Recommendations have not been developed for all of the risk groups initially considered owing to a lack of evidence (see Section 4.2). Additional risk groups may be considered for screening based on the criteria set out in the key principles in Section 7.

The evidence is summarized in the GRADE table in *Annex 1* in this document, and in the GRADE tables for specific risk groups and Decision tables in the supporting material available at www.who.int/tb/tbscreening.

8.1 Strong recommendations

Recommendation 1

Household contacts and other close contacts should be systematically screened for active TB.

(Strong recommendation, very low-quality evidence)

Remarks
While the quality of the direct evidence is low for the benefit of TB screening for close contacts of someone with TB, the Guideline Development Group placed high value on ensuring early diagnosis in this risk group, which has a high likelihood of having undetected TB and a high risk of poor health outcomes in the absence of early diagnosis and treatment; these considerations are especially important for young children. This recommendation is fully consistent with recommendations in the previous WHO guideline (*Recommendations for investigating the contacts of persons with infectious tuberculosis in low- and middle-income countries*).[11]

See the guidelines on contact investigation[11] for details on:
- definitions of "close contact", "household contact", and "index case";
- prioritizing index cases;
- choosing diagnostic tools for people who are at risk of multidrug-resistant TB (MDR-TB) and people who are HIV-positive or have a high risk of being HIV-positive;
- treating latent TB infection;

- offering HIV counselling and testing as part of the investigation of contacts;
- operational aspects of investigating contacts, including choosing an approach (for example, by inviting a contact to attend a health facility or by visiting the household),the timing of the visit and the possibility of repeating screening.

When resources are limited, a decision should be made about which index cases to follow up with contact investigation. Contact investigation should always be done when the index case has any of the following characteristics: sputum smear-positive pulmonary TB, proven or suspected MDR-TB or extensively drug-resistant TB, is a person living with HIV or is a child younger than 5 years. In addition, resources permitting, contact investigation for household contacts and close contacts may be performed for all other index cases with pulmonary TB.

Section 9 presents options for algorithms for adults and children. The choice of algorithm depends on the situation in the country and the availability of resources.

People identified through screening and suspected of having active TB but in whom active TB has not been diagnosed should be informed about the importance of seeking medical care if TB symptoms continue, emerge, re-emerge or worsen. If possible, repeat testing for TB should be offered.

Children who are younger than 5 years and who are household contacts or close contacts of someone with TB and who, after screening and appropriate diagnostic evaluation (if indicated), are judged not to have active TB should be treated for presumed latent TB infection according to WHO's guidelines (see WHO's contact-investigation guidelines[11] and *Guidance for national tuberculosis programmes on the management of tuberculosis in children*[72]).

In settings with a high prevalence of HIV all household contacts and close contacts should be offered HIV counselling and testing for HIV. When an index case is a person living with HIV, all household contacts should be offered HIV counselling and testing for HIV. All household contacts and close contacts who have symptoms compatible with active TB should be offered HIV counselling and testing for HIV as part of their clinical evaluation. People living with HIV who are household contacts or close contacts and who, after an appropriate clinical evaluation, are found not to have active TB should be treated for presumed latent TB infection following WHO's *Guidelines for intensified tuberculosis case-finding and isoniazid preventive therapy for people living with HIV in resource-constrained settings*[10] and *Recommendations for investigating the contacts of persons with infectious tuberculosis in low- and middle-income countries*.[11]

Contacts should have a nutrition screening and assessment as part of the investigation. If malnutrition is identified, it should be managed according to WHO's recommendations. For further details, see WHO's guidelines on nutritional care and support for people with TB.[73]

For a review of the evidence, see WHO's guideline on contact investigation,[11] the summary GRADE table in *Annex 1* in this document, and the GRADE table for specific risk groups and the Decision table that are available as supporting material at www.who.int/tb/tbscreening.

Recommendation 2

People living with HIV should be systematically screened for active TB at each visit to a health facility.

(Strong recommendation, very low-quality evidence)

Remarks
While the quality of the direct evidence is very low for the benefit of TB screening in people living with HIV, the Guideline Development Group placed high value on ensuring that TB is diagnosed early in this risk group, which has a high likelihood of having undetected TB and a high risk of poor health outcomes in the absence of early diagnosis and treatment. This recommendation is fully consistent with previous WHO's *Guidelines for intensified tuberculosis case-finding and isoniazid preventive therapy for people living with HIV in resource-constrained settings*,[10] and these guidelines provide further details on diagnostic evaluation, operational aspects of screening, and monitoring and evaluating screening.

68 The following screening options are recommended in WHO's guidelines on intensified case-finding in people living with HIV:[10]

- people living with HIV in resource-constrained settings should be screened with a clinical algorithm, and those who report any one of the symptoms of current cough, fever, weight loss or night sweats should be evaluated for TB and other diseases;
- chest radiography can be considered to augment symptom-based screening in settings with a high prevalence of TB among people living with HIV.

The use of chest radiography is often accompanied by significant concerns about costs, workload, infrastructure and the availability of qualified staff. Therefore, it may not be possible to use chest radiography in many settings.

Persons living with HIV whose screening test is positive should have an Xpert MTB/RIF test as a primary diagnostic test.[74]

People who do not report any one of the symptoms of current cough, fever, weight loss or night sweats are unlikely to have active TB, and should be offered treatment for presumed latent TB infection.

For a review of the evidence, see WHO's guidelines on intensified case-finding in people living with HIV[10] and the Decision table in the supporting material available at www.who.int/tb/tbscreening.

Recommendation 3

Current and former workers in workplaces with silica exposure should be systematically screened for active TB.

(Strong recommendation, low-quality evidence)

Remarks
While the quality of the direct evidence is very low for the benefit of TB screening in employees in workplaces where they are exposed to silica, the Guideline Development Group placed high value on ensuring that TB is diagnosed early in this risk group, which has a high likelihood of having undetected TB as well as other pulmonary diseases that may be detected through screening.

Section 9 presents options for algorithms for screening and diagnosis. The choice of algorithm depends on the epidemiology of TB and the availability of resources.

Contacts in the workplace should be investigated when a new case of TB is diagnosed (see Recommendation 1).

There is limited evidence on the effectiveness of different screening intervals. The panel suggests that the screening interval should be no longer than 12 months if possible, while an interval shorter than 12 months may be more beneficial.

People identified through screening and suspected of having active TB but in whom active TB has not been diagnosed and treated should be informed about the importance of seeking medical care if TB symptoms continue, emerge, re-emerge or worsen. If possible, repeat testing for TB should be offered.

HIV counselling and testing should be offered to all people with suspected TB.[10,75] In settings with a high prevalence of HIV, counselling and testing for HIV may be offered to all people screened for TB.

To the extent possible, TB screening should be combined with screening for other diseases and health-promotion activities, and with efforts to improve working conditions (especially by reducing exposure to silica) and living conditions.

During employment, screening should be considered to be the responsibility of the employer, and countries may have occupational health and safety legislation that addresses this.

For a review of the evidence, see the summary GRADE table in *Annex 1* in this document, and the GRADE table for specific risk groups and the Decision table in the supporting material available at www.who.int/tb/tbscreening.

8.2 Conditional recommendations

Recommendation 4

Systematic screening for active TB should be considered in prisons and other penitentiary institutions.

(Conditional recommendation, very low-quality evidence)

Remarks
The panel did not reach consensus on this recommendation. About 40% of the panel voted in favour of a strong recommendation for screening in prisons and other penitentiary institutions in settings where the TB prevalence in the general population is more than 100/100 000 population, and for a conditional recommendation for settings where the prevalence is less than 100/100 000. The majority of the panel voted for one conditional recommendation for all settings while stating that screening in prisons should be prioritized in settings where the prevalence of TB in the general population or in the prison population, or both, is high; where the incarceration rate is high; where there is a high prevalence of HIV or MDR-TB ; or where living conditions in prisons and other penitentiary institutions are poor.

It may not be possible to implement this recommendation in resource-constrained settings.

People in prisons and other penitentiary institutions who are eligible for screening include both prisoners and prison staff. A prisoner is anyone held in a criminal justice facility or correctional facility during the investigation of a crime, anyone awaiting trial and anyone who has been sentenced.

When starting screening, it is important to ensure that good treatment and case management, as well as effective mechanisms for continuing treatment after transfer or release, are in place. For recommendations on and operational aspects associated with TB care and prevention in prisons and other penitentiary institutions, see *Guidelines for the control of tuberculosis in prisons.*[12] However, even if TB management practices are suboptimal, screening may be initiated to assess the burden of undetected TB among inmates and thus provide a rationale for strengthening general diagnostic and treatment services for TB, as well as implementing measures to improve infection control and living conditions.

Section 9 presents options for screening and diagnosis. There is no evidence about the effectiveness of using different timings for screening and different screening intervals. The panel believes that screening in prisons and other penitentiary institutions should always include screening when a person enters a detention facility, and that annual screening should be considered if resources permit. Exit screening, for people leaving detention, should be considered when possible and when treatment and follow up after release can be ensured.

Contacts should be investigated whenever a new case is detected (see Recommendation 1).

People who develop symptoms suggestive of TB after the initial screening should have easy access to diagnostic testing. People identified through screening and suspected of having active TB but in whom active TB has not been diagnosed should be informed about the importance of seeking medical care if TB symptoms continue, emerge, re-emerge or worsen.

HIV counselling and testing should be offered to all people suspected of having TB.[10,76] In settings with a high prevalence of HIV, counselling and testing for HIV may be offered to all people screened for TB.

Screening in prisons should be combined with efforts to improve living conditions and infection control (see guidelines on infection control in prisons and guidelines on control in other congregate settings).[76,12] If possible, TB screening in prisons and other penitentiary institutions should be combined with screening for other diseases and health-promotion activities targeting this group.

For a review of the evidence, see the summary GRADE table in *Annex 1* in this document, and the GRADE table for specific risk groups and the Decision table in the supporting material available at www.who.int/tb/tbscreening.

Recommendation 5

Systematic screening for active TB should be considered in people with an untreated fibrotic lesion seen on chest X-ray.

(Conditional recommendation, very low-quality evidence)

Remarks

It may not be possible to implement this recommendation in resource-constrained settings.

Screening may be done by inviting members of this group to a TB facility or general health facility. People with an untreated fibrotic lesion seen on a chest radiograph may be identified when other risk groups are screened for TB.

Section 9 presents options for screening and diagnosis. There is no evidence about the effectiveness of different screening intervals or the total duration of follow up. The panel believes that the interval and duration should be guided by feasibility.

People who are not diagnosed with active TB should be informed about the importance seeking medical care if TB symptoms emerge.

For a review of the evidence, see the summary GRADE table in *Annex 1* in this document, and the GRADE table for specific risk groups and the Decision table in the supporting material available at www.who.int/tb/tbscreening.

Recommendation 6

In settings where the TB prevalence in the general population is 100/100 000 population or higher, systematic screening for active TB should be considered among people who are seeking health care or who are in health care and who belong to selected risk groups (see below).

(Conditional recommendation, very low-quality evidence)

Remarks

This recommendation concerns interventions that should be undertaken in addition to passive case-finding – that is, in addition to properly triaging people seeking care who have a cough, which should be done in all settings, [77] and which it is particularly important to implement rigorously among people who have risk factors for TB.

It may not be possible to implement this recommendation in resource-constrained settings.

Risk groups should be prioritized based on their risk of TB, the risk of poor treatment outcomes if diagnosis is delayed and the size of the risk group in a given setting. People who are living with HIV, people who have had recent close contact with a person who has TB, people who have silicosis or have a fibrotic lesion identified by chest radiography should be screened for TB as described in recommendations 1, 2, 3 and 5. Other risk groups that should be considered for screening are listed in *Table 9*; the table also presents data on the risk of TB and the risk of poor treatment outcomes. Other risk groups – such as people with malignancies and other disorders that compromise their immune system, and people receiving immunomodulatory therapies – may also be prioritized, depending on the local epidemiology and capacity of the health system. Screening for latent TB infection and providing preventive treatment in people starting on immunosuppressive treatment is not covered by this recommendation.

Table 9. **Risk of TB and poor health outcomes in clinical risk groups**

Risk factor	Risk of TB	Health outcomes related to risk factor
Underweight (BMI <18.5)	Pooled relative risk estimate from meta-analysis: 3.2 (95% CI, 3.1–3.3)[78]	Increased risk of death and TB relapse; systematic reviews, no pooled estimate[79,66]
Gastrectomy or jejunoileal bypass	No pooled estimate Gastrectomy: relative risk range, 2–5. Bypass: relative risk range, 27–63[68,,80]	Increased risk of death associated with undernutrition (see "Underweight"), but no published data specifically on gastrectomy or jejunoileal bypass
Diabetes mellitus	Pooled relative risk estimate from systematic review: 3.1 (95% CI, 2.3–4.3)[81]	Pooled relative risk of TB treatment failure or death from systematic review: 1.69 (95% CI, 1.36–2.12) and relapse: 3.89 (95% CI, 2.43–6.23)[82]
Alcohol dependence	Pooled relative risk estimate from systematic review: 2.9 (95% CI, 1.9–4.6)[83]	Higher risk of TB treatment failure and relapse and death during treatment; systematic review, no pooled estimate[84]
Tobacco smoking	Pooled relative risk estimate from systematic review: 2.0 (95% CI, 1.6–2.5)[85]	Increased risk of death; systematic review, no pooled estimate[86]
Chronic renal failure or haemodialysis	No pooled estimate; relative risk range, 10-25[68,81]	Increased risk of death; systematic review, no pooled estimate[86]
Intravenous drug use	No pooled estimate;[17] increased risk probably due to high prevalence of other risk factors, such as HIV	Increased risk of death; systematic review, no pooled estimate[66]
Solid organ transplantation	No pooled estimate; relative risk range, 20–74[81]	No published data
Old age	Not established; prevalence surveys report increased risk with age[27,28]	Increased risk of death; systematic review, no pooled estimate[66]
Previously treated TB	High incidence of TB due to relapse and reinfection;[87,88,89] no systematic review	Retreatment cases have higher risk of poor outcomes and higher risk of MDR-TB
Pregnancy	Not established[90]	Infants of mothers with TB have increased risks of premature birth and perinatal death;[91,9293] pregnant women with TB are more likely to have complications during pregnancy; initiating TB treatment is associated with better maternal and infant outcomes than late initiation[94,95,96,97.98]

BMI, body mass index; CI, confidence interval; MDR-TB, multidrug-resistant TB.

People identified through screening and suspected of having active TB but who are not diagnosed with active TB should be informed about the importance of seeking medical care if TB symptoms continue, emerge, re-emerge or worsen. If possible, repeat testing for TB should be offered.

Section 9 presents options for screening and diagnosis. The choice of algorithm for screening and diagnosis depends on the background epidemiology of TB, the risk group and the availability of resources. The use of chest radiography in pregnant women poses no significant risk,[99] but national guidelines for the use of radiography during pregnancy should be followed.

There is no evidence about the appropriate interval between screenings. The Guideline Development Group believes that screening should be offered if it has not been done during the previous 12 months. However, this interval is arbitrary, and a different interval may be applied depending on the risk group, the availability of resources and the feasibility.

HIV counselling and testing should be offered to all people suspected of having TB.[10,75] In settings with a high prevalence of HIV, counselling and testing for HIV may be offered to all people screened for TB.

Risk groups should be targeted within the clinic where they are managed – for example, pregnant women may be targeted at the antenatal clinic, and people with diabetes may be targeted by the endocrinology department.

Screening people with diabetes for TB should be combined with reciprocal screening for diabetes in people with TB; for additional information, see the *Collaborative framework for care and control of tuberculosis and diabetes.*[14]

In respiratory clinics, screening smokers or people with chronic obstructive pulmonary disease for TB can be combined with reciprocal screening for smoking and respiratory conditions in people with TB; for additional information see the *Practical approach to lung health*[100] and the monograph by WHO and the International Union Against Tuberculosis and Lung Disease on TB and tobacco control.[101]

Screening for TB in people with alcohol-use disorders or other drug-use disorders can be combined with HIV screening in drug users, and can also be reciprocated with screening for alcohol use and drug use in people with TB; for additional information see the *Policy guidelines for collaborative TB and HIV services for injecting and other drug users: an integrated approach.*[17]

In health facilities, screening for active TB should be offered to health-care staff and combined with other infection-control interventions; for additional information see guidelines on infection control in health facilities[77].

For a review of the evidence, see the summary GRADE table in *Annex 1* in this document, and the Decision table in the supporting material available at www.who.int/tb/tbscreening.

Recommendation 7
(a) Systematic screening for active TB may be considered for geographically defined subpopulations with extremely high levels of undetected TB (1% prevalence or higher).

(b) Systematic screening for active TB may be considered also for other subpopulations that have very poor access to health care, such as people living in urban slums, homeless people, people living in remote areas with poor access to health care, and other vulnerable or marginalized groups including some indigenous populations, migrants and refugees.

(Conditional recommendation, very low-quality evidence)

Remarks
It may not be possible to implement this recommendation in resource-constrained settings owing to its high costs and considerable requirements for human resources.

The list of potential target groups in Recommendation 7b is not exhaustive, and they may include other groups with a high risk of TB or who have poor access to high-quality TB services (see *Table 1* and *Table 6*).

Community screening can be done by:
- inviting people to attend screening at a mobile facility or a fixed facility. Invitations may target specifically people with the highest prevalence of TB within a given risk group, including people living with HIV, those who

have had recent close contact with someone who has TB and people with symptoms of TB;
- going door to door to screen households; or
- systematically screen individuals in shelters, refugee camps and other specific locations.

The intensity of the approach used for community screening will have an impact on final yield; and more intensive approaches require more resources. The primary goal of screening in these groups is to improve individual health outcomes. Only one randomized controlled study has evaluated the impact of TB screening on transmission. It provided moderate-quality evidence that community screening aiming at increasing awareness of TB symptoms and making it easy to access smear microscopy did not increase case notifications, reduce the prevalence of undiagnosed TB or reduce TB transmission. The impact on transmission is uncertain when a more sensitive screening approach is used (see Section 5.1).

Section 9 presents options for screening and diagnosis. The choice of algorithm for screening and diagnosis depends on the epidemiology of TB in the targeted group, the screening approach used and the availability of resources.

There is no evidence about the effectiveness of different screening intervals. The Guideline Development Group believes that the interval should be guided by feasibility.

People identified through screening and suspected of having active TB but who are not diagnosed with active TB should be informed about the importance of seeking medical care if TB symptoms continue, emerge, re-emerge or worsen. If possible, repeat testing for TB should be offered.

HIV counselling and testing should be offered to all people with suspected TB.[10,75] In settings with a high prevalence of HIV, counselling and testing for HIV may be offered to all people screened for TB.

To the extent possible, community screening should be combined with screening for other diseases or risk factors, and with health-promotion activities or social support.

When screening is done in refugee camps and among displaced populations, consult *Tuberculosis care and control in refugee and displaced populations* for recommendations on TB management and operational considerations.[13]

Pre-migration screening of people other than refugees – for example a visa applicant from a high-burden country seeking to migrate to a low-burden country – requires special consideration: the migrants may be considered to be members of a high-risk group by the country to which they are moving but normally they are not considered to be at high risk in their country of origin. This group should be prioritized for screening based on the principles set out in Section 7.[102]

For a review of the evidence, see the summary GRADE table in *Annex 1* in this document, and the GRADE tables for specific risk groups and the Decision table in the supporting material available at www.who.int/tb/tbscreening.

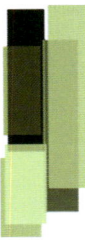

9. Algorithms for screening and diagnosis

The algorithms for screening and diagnosis were developed using the GRADE tables from Review 2 on the sensitivity and specificity of different screening tools (*Annex II*) and the modelled yield of different algorithms at different levels of TB prevalence (see supporting material available at www.who.int/tb/tbscreening). *Annex III* includes flow charts for the different algorithms, and provides the estimated yield and predictive values for each.

The options for initial screening include symptom screening (screening either for cough lasting longer than 2 weeks, or screening for any symptom compatible with TB, including cough of any duration, haemoptysis, weight loss, fever or night sweats) or screening with chest radiography. If symptom screening is used as the initial screening test, chest radiography can be used as the second screening to further improve the pretest probability of the subsequent diagnostic test, and to reduce the number of people who need to undergo further diagnostic evaluation.

As part of the initial screening, each algorithm includes a step to identify people living with HIV; people who are HIV-positive should be assessed by following the *Guidelines for intensified tuberculosis case-finding and isoniazid preventive therapy for people living with HIV in resource-constrained setting.*[10] Screening can therefore be enhanced by combining screening for TB with screening for HIV.

The following algorithms for screening and diagnosis should be considered.

9.1 Screening adults and children aged 10 years or older

Algorithms 1 a–d (see Annex III): *This option includes an interview about TB symptoms and HIV status. All people with cough lasting longer than 2 weeks should be investigated for TB. Chest radiography should be considered as a second screening for people who have had a cough lasting longer than 2*

weeks; and people with an abnormal chest radiograph suggestive of TB[iii]
should be evaluated for TB. For people known to be HIV-positive, see the
Guidelines for intensified tuberculosis case-finding and isoniazid preventive
therapy for people living with HIV in resource-constrained settings .[10]

Algorithms 2 a–d (see Annex III): *This option includes an interview about*
TB symptoms and HIV status. Further investigation for TB should be done for
persons with any of the following symptoms: cough of any duration,
haemoptysis, weight loss, fever or night sweats. Chest radiography should be
considered for the second screening for people who screened positive when
asked about symptoms; and people with an abnormal chest radiograph
suggestive of TB should be evaluated for TB. For people known to be HIV-
positive, see the guidelines on intensified case-finding for people living with
HIV.[10]

Algorithms 3 a–b (see Annex III): *This option includes chest radiography and*
an interview about HIV status. Persons with an abnormal chest radiograph
suggestive of TB should be evaluated for TB. For persons known to be HIV-
positive, see the guidelines on intensified case-finding for people living with
HIV.[10]

Each algorithm for adults includes options for the initial diagnostic testing of
people whose screening test is positive: either sputum-smear microscopy[iv] or
a rapid molecular test that has been demonstrated to have high accuracy for
both smear-positive and smear-negative pulmonary TB, such as the Xpert
MTB/RIF test (or any rapid test recommended by WHO in the future that has
the same or better accuracy[49]). Positive or negative diagnostic results may
require a repeat test or further diagnostic evaluation using culture, drug-
susceptibility testing, clinical assessment, or some combination of these.
Culture is the gold standard of diagnostic testing for TB. However, in these
algorithms it is not considered for use as an initial diagnostic test because it
demands more resources and requires a much longer wait for results (2–6
weeks) than the Xpert MTB/RIF test and sputum-smear microscopy, both of
which can provide final results in less than 1 day. Where resources permit,

---

[iii] Chest radiographs suggestive of TB may be separated into those that are
suggestive of active TB and those that are suggestive of either active or inactive TB.
[iv] This refers to conventional light microscopy used to examine direct smears stained
with Ziehl–Neelsen (with or without specific sputum-processing methods) or
fluorescence microscopy (including microscopy with light-emitting diodes). •

and where the health system has sufficient capacity to ensure that patients are followed up after culture results are available, culture may be used in parallel with or after testing with the Xpert MTB/RIF or sputum-smear microscopy. Culture with drug-susceptibility testing should be done according to the guidelines for diagnosing drug-resistant TB.[16]

The choice of algorithm depends on the risk group being assessed, the prevalence of TB, the availability of resources and the feasibility (see remarks).

Remarks for all algorithms for screening adults and children aged 10 years or older
- Especially when the prevalence of TB is moderate or low, it is critical to ensure that the algorithm used has high specificity in order to avoid a low positive predictive value of the final diagnosis, and hence avoid a high proportion of false-positive TB cases. At a TB prevalence of 0.5% in the screened population, all of the algorithms have a positive predictive value of less than 75% when clinical diagnosis is used (with chest radiography and clinical evaluation) for all or some of those with a negative result from their initial diagnostic test. Even when clinical diagnosis is not considered, the positive predictive value is below 80% for all but one algorithm (algorithm 1d: screening for cough lasting longer than 2 weeks followed by screening with chest radiography and testing with Xpert MTB/RIF). Special attention must be paid to the quality of diagnostic procedures and clinical assessment when TB prevalence in the screened population is moderate to low. If the positive predictive value is low then repeat tests may be necessary as well as a confirmatory culture.

- When the TB prevalence is 1% or higher, the positive predictive value is higher than 80% for some algorithms (1b–d, 2d and 3b, not considering clinical diagnosis), but diagnostic quality must still be optimized.

- Especially in groups with a high risk of severe negative effects from missed or delayed diagnosis and treatment, it is important to use an algorithm that has very high sensitivity, although this often leads to lower specificity. The risk of a false-positive diagnosis of active TB must also be considered in these groups. However, the benefits of providing early treatment may outweigh the risks of treating a false-positive case of TB. Particularly in persons who may be eligible for treatment for latent TB infection (such as contacts younger than 5 years and people living with HIV) it is more important to rule out active TB than to avoid a false-positive diagnosis of active TB. Sensitivity is therefore more important than specificity for such persons.

- In many settings high-quality chest radiography and people qualified to read chest radiographs may not be available. The Xpert MTB/RIF test may not be available in many settings. It may not be possible to implement the Xpert MTB/RIF test or chest radiography in all settings. When this is the case, the priority should be to introduce these tests into regular diagnostic services before considering introducing screening.

- Individuals known to have TB or suspected of having TB and who are at high risk of MDR-TB should always have an Xpert MTB/RIF test as their primary diagnostic test, if it is available. This group includes persons suspected of having pulmonary TB and considered to be at risk of harbouring MDR-TB bacilli. These risk groups should be defined by national policies or as defined in WHO's *Guidelines for the programmatic management of drug-resistant tuberculosis;*[16] the groups include persons who have been treated with anti-TB medicines and in whom pulmonary TB has again been diagnosed – that is, all retreatment categories (failure, default, relapse).

- When the prevalence of rifampicin resistance in the screened population is less than 10%, an Xpert MTB/RIF result that is positive for rifampicin resistance should be confirmed by conventional drug-susceptibility testing or line probe assay.[74]

- All algorithms include an interview about HIV status. Offering HIV counselling and testing should be considered an integral part of TB screening, especially in settings with a high prevalence of HIV, in order to both improve the performance of the screening algorithm and contribute to the early diagnosis, treatment and care of people with HIV.

- If it is available, an Xpert MTB/RIF test should be given as the primary diagnostic test to all persons living with HIV who have signs or symptoms of TB, to persons who are seriously ill and are suspected of having TB regardless of their HIV status, and to persons whose HIV status is unknown but who present with strong clinical evidence of HIV infection in settings where the prevalence of HIV is high.[75]

- Children aged 10 years and older should be screened with the same algorithm that is used for adults. No published study has specifically assessed the sensitivity and specificity of screening algorithms used for children and adolescents who are not contacts of people with TB. The Guideline Development Group believes that the screening algorithm for adults is likely to have similar accuracy in children aged 10 years and older.

Remarks for Algorithm 1
- Screening for cough lasting longer than 2 weeks has a low sensitivity.

- The sensitivity of the whole algorithm is further reduced when sputum-smear microscopy is used for diagnosis. The sensitivity of sputum-smear microscopy varies with the quality of smear preparation and reading as well as with the proportion in the tested population of smear-positive TB cases out of total culture-positive cases. Sensitivity can be improved with various sputum-processing methods and with fluorescence microscopy, but such methods may reduce specificity.[50]

- The specificity of sputum-smear microscopy varies depending on the case definition, the prevalence of nontubercular mycobacteria, the gold standard used for assessment, and the quality of slide preparation and reading. When using WHO 's case definition of identifying one positive smear out of two, the pooled specificity for conventional smear microscopy is 98% (95% confidence interval, 93– 99%), and it may be lower when different methods are used to improve the sensitivity of sputum-smear microscopy.[104,,51,103]

- A 1% reduction in specificity from 99% to 98% leads to about double the number of false-positive cases when the prevalence in the screened group is low.

- False-positive diagnoses caused by inappropriate smear preparation or reading, contamination or operational errors can be reduced by repeating tests for those who test positive or by doing alternative confirmatory diagnostic tests. Therefore, when the prevalence of TB is low, additional testing should be considered.

- Because sputum-smear microscopy has low sensitivity, additional diagnostic evaluation is often required for persons whose test results are negative, especially when the prevalence of TB is high (which reduces the negative predictive value). The specificity of diagnosis of smear-negative TB based on chest radiography and clinical evaluation is low (about 94% – that is, five times as many false-positive cases occur when compared with a test that has 99% specificity); this leads to a high number of false-positive cases if a large proportion of people with negative sputum-smear microscopy undergo clinical diagnosis. At up to 2% prevalence of TB in the screened population, the positive predictive value for all algorithms is less than 75% when sputum-smear microscopy is used as the initial diagnostic test and where clinical diagnosis is considered for those who test negative by sputum-smear microscopy. It is therefore critical to optimize the accuracy of sputum-smear microscopy and clinical diagnosis, particularly when the prevalence in the screened population is less than 2%. If good-quality culture is available, it can be used to improve the specificity of the final diagnosis.

- The Xpert MTB/RIF[v] test has higher sensitivity than sputum-smear microscopy, but the overall sensitivity of the algorithm is limited by the low sensitivity of screening for cough lasting longer than 2 weeks.

- The likelihood of TB among people with cough lasting longer than 2 weeks and who have a negative result on the Xpert MTB/RIF test (1 – negative predictive value) is low (0.6% at 1% prevalence, and 1.2% at 2% prevalence). Nevertheless, repeat testing with the Xpert MTB/RIF or further diagnostic evaluation and testing with culture may be required for people among whom there is a high clinical suspicion for TB.

- Using the Xpert MTB/RIF test as a follow-on test for persons whose sputum-smear microscopy was negative, improves both the sensitivity and specificity of the diagnosis of smear-negative TB when compared with clinical diagnosis. However, if the Xpert MTB/RIF test is available at the point of care (or sputum transportation can be organized for

---

[v] This is true for any other test with the same or better accuracy than the Xpert MTB/RIF, including any rapid tests endorsed by WHO in the future.

everyone who is tested), then ideally it should be used as the initial test instead of sputum-smear microscopy. At a 1% prevalence of TB in the screened population (when screening for cough lasting longer than 2 weeks gives a pretest probability for sputum-smear microscopy of 6%), 94% of people who are positive by screening will be negative by sputum-smear microscopy. Therefore, the number of Xpert MTB/RIF tests will be reduced only marginally by using sputum-smear microscopy first, and 94% of those whose screening is positive, but who are smear-negative, will be tested by both sputum-smear microscopy and Xpert MTB/RIF. Moreover, the total number of false-positive cases will be higher if sputum-smear microscopy is used first. When the Xpert MTB/RIF test is available only through referral (for example, to tertiary level), it can be used as part of a further diagnostic evaluation among people who are sputum smear-negative and who have been judged to have a high likelihood of TB.

- The specificity of the Xpert MTB/RIF test is high (99%). However, at 0.5% prevalence the positive predictive value is only 75%. Repeat testing and further diagnostic evaluation can reduce the number of false-positive cases.

- Using chest radiography as a the second screening test after positive symptom screening improves specificity significantly and reduces sensitivity only marginally.

- A second screen with chest radiography followed by sputum-smear microscopy yields not only a high proportion of false-negative cases but also a high proportion of false-positive cases. Furthermore, persons who have both cough lasting longer than 2 weeks and an abnormality on chest radiography suggestive of TB, but who are sputum-smear negative, normally need further clinical evaluation since the negative predictive value is low. This further reduces the overall specificity and generates additional false-positive cases. Therefore, screening with chest radiography should ideally be followed by testing with Xpert MTB/RIF which has higher negative predictive value as well as higher positive predictive value than sputum-smear microscopy.

- Using chest radiography as a second screening test reduces the number of Xpert MTB/RIF tests in those whose screening was positive when compared with using only cough lasting longer than 2 weeks. For example, at 1% prevalence the number of required Xpert MTB/RIF tests per 1 true case is 9 compared with 17 Xpert MTB/RIF tests when chest radiography is not used for the second screening.

- Screening with chest radiography may be done for abnormalities suggestive of active TB, or for abnormalities suggestive of either active or inactive TB.

Remarks for Algorithm 2
- Algorithm 2 has higher overall sensitivity than Algorithm 1 (71% compared with 32% when Xpert MTB/RIF testing is used for diagnosis). However, it generates a larger number of persons with positive screening results, and therefore requires more resources than Algorithm 1.

- Algorithm 2 has lower specificity than Algorithm 1. At 1% prevalence, the positive predictive value for a positive Xpert MTB/RIF test is 69%, and it is only 40% for positive sputum-smear microscopy, whereas Algorithm 1 has positive predictive values of 85% for a positive Xpert MTB/RIF and 67% for a positive sputum smear. Algorithm 2 should be used for risk groups where a high sensitivity is important, and for whom the negative consequences of a false-positive diagnosis are less severe. When high sensitivity is required, the Xpert MTB/RIF test is the preferred diagnostic test. The same principles for improving the specificity of the final diagnosis as described for Algorithm 1 apply to Algorithm 2.

- Similar to Algorithm 1, using chest radiography for the second screening in Algorithm 2 improves the specificity and the positive predictive value of the final diagnosis significantly; it also reduces the number of Xpert MTB/RIF tests required, while reducing sensitivity only marginally.

- Screening with chest radiography may be done for abnormalities suggestive of active TB, or for abnormalities suggestive of either active or inactive TB.

Remarks for Algorithm 3
- Algorithm 3 is the most sensitive of the algorithms, especially when the Xpert MTB/RIF test is used for diagnosis. However, it demands the most resources.

- Using chest radiography for screening followed by sputum-smear microscopy yields not only a high proportion of false-negative cases but also a high proportion of false-positive cases. A large proportion of people who are positive when screened by chest radiography are likely to undergo clinical diagnosis, which further increases the number of false-positive cases.

- Using the Xpert MTB/RIF test for diagnosis increases the number of true cases diagnosed, and reduces the number of false-positive cases when compared with using sputum-smear microscopy for diagnosis. The Xpert MTB/RIF test is the preferred diagnostic test for use after screening with chest radiography.

- Screening with chest radiography can be done either to identify only abnormalities typically associated with active TB or to identify abnormalities suggestive of either active or inactive TB. A few people with abnormalities suggestive of inactive TB in fact have active TB. Therefore, identifying abnormalities suggestive of either active or inactive TB is more sensitive but less specific than identifying only abnormalities associated with active TB. For recommendations on interpreting chest radiographs and practical advice on using chest radiography, see WHO's *Tuberculosis prevalence surveys: a handbook.*[100]

- Using chest radiography to screen for abnormalities that are suggestive of either active or inactive TB is the most sensitive of the screening options in the algorithms when it is combined with an Xpert MTB/RIF test for diagnosis; this screening should be considered for risk groups in which it is critical not to miss TB. However, the positive predictive value must be considered. At 1% prevalence the positive predictive value is 78% with an Xpert MTB/RIF test for diagnosis, and at 0.5% prevalence it is 64% . Further diagnostic verification may be required.

- At a prevalence less than 0.5%, using chest radiography to screen for abnormalities suggestive of active TB followed by an Xpert MTB/RIF test yields 20% false-positive cases (positive predictive value, 79 at 0.5% prevalence) unless further diagnostic verification is done. Culture or careful diagnostic assessment, or both, are necessary for persons who are positive by Xpert MTB/RIF testing, especially when the TB prevalence is less than 0.5%. Using Algorithm 1 with chest radiography for the second screening has a higher positive predictive value (88% at a prevalence of 0.5%), and it should be considered as an alternative. However, the sensitivity will be much lower than when using chest radiography as the initial screening test.

9.2   Screening children younger than 10 years

Screening children who are living with HIV or who are contacts of someone with TB
- *For children who are living with HIV or who are contacts of someone with TB, symptom-based screening should be done to identify those with cough, fever, weight loss or fatigue of any duration; children with any symptom should be investigated for TB.*
- *For children who are living with HIV or who are contacts of someone with TB, chest radiography may be added to the initial screening. Children with any symptom or a chest radiograph with an abnormality suggestive of TB should be investigated to determine whether they have TB.*

Screening children in situations other than as part of contact investigation or screening among people living with HIV
- *For children who are younger than 10 years and who are screened in situations other than as part of a contact investigation or screening for people living with HIV, an interview should be done to determine whether the child is known to be HIV-positive or has had recent contact with someone who has TB, in either case the algorithm options for children younger than 10 years who are living with HIV or who are contacts of someone with TB apply.*

Remarks on screening algorithms for children
- For diagnosing TB in children whose screening is positive, see *Guidance for national tuberculosis programmes on the management of tuberculosis in children.*[73]

- Children younger than 5 years who are contacts of someone with TB and all children who are known to be HIV-positive should be treated for latent TB infection if active TB has been ruled out.[10,11 72]

- The finding of hilar adenopathy by chest radiography in an asymptomatic child may represent a contained TB infection, and the child may not require treatment for active TB.

- Using chest radiography as a screening tool requires the ability to subsequently conduct a careful clinical assessment, with follow up if required, to establish a diagnosis of active TB disease. High-quality chest radiography, staff qualified to read chest radiographs, and specialists who can conduct additional clinical assessments may not be available in all setting. In resource-constrained settings, it may not be possible to follow the algorithm that uses chest radiography.

- No study has assessed screening algorithms for children aged 5–15 years or for children younger than 5 years who are not contacts of someone with TB or who are not HIV-positive. However, the Guideline Development Group considers that symptom screening as well as screening with chest radiography in children who are younger than 10 years is likely to have very low specificity, since pulmonary TB would be a relatively rare cause of lower respiratory symptoms and signs, which are common in this age group. A large number of young children who do not have TB would have additional investigations if young children were systematically screened as part of a general screening programme. Furthermore, most confirmatory diagnostic tests for TB have lower accuracy in children than in adults, and the final diagnosis (including clinical assessment) would be uncertain among many of those who had additional evaluations. This would likely result in not only a high number of false-positive cases but also a high number of false-negative cases. The Guideline Development Group thus judges that there is risk of doing more harm than benefit by screening children who are younger than 10 years, except to identify children who are known to be HIV-positive or have had recent contact with someone who has TB.

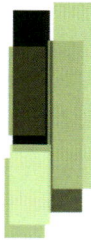

10. Monitoring and evaluation

10.1 Proposed indicators

The following indicators should be considered for each targeted risk group:
1. the number of people eligible for screening;
2. the number of people screened (considering the first screening and second screening separately, if applicable);
3. the proportion of those eligible for screening who were screened;
4. the number of people with suspected TB who were identified;
5. the number of people undergoing diagnostic investigation;
6. the number of people diagnosed with TB by type of TB;
7. the proportion of those undergoing diagnostic investigation who have TB;
8. the number needed to screen to detect one case of TB;
9. the proportion of initial defaulters (that is, the number of people diagnosed with TB who do NOT start treatment divided by number of people diagnosed with TB);
10. the treatment success rate and death rate (using standard cohort analyses).

Additional disaggregation may be done – for example, by age and sex – but this requires that more detailed data are collected for each individual who is screened.

The uptake of screening (the proportion of those eligible for screening who are actually screened) in a risk group can be assessed only if the size of the target group has been well defined. It is normally possible to obtain the relevant information for screening conducted within health facilities, closed settings (such as prisons) and through contact investigations. However, it is often difficult to obtain this information from outreach screening programmes – for example, when screening is done in the community – although the estimated population size of a targeted community may be used to obtain a rough estimate of the eligible population.

10.2   Routines for recording and reporting

In order to obtain the required information for the indicators described above, a TB recording and reporting system needs to include:

- a log of the number of people screened in each risk group. A special register with individual-level information for each person screened may be used to obtain more refined data about subcategories of persons within a risk group. Collecting these data is resource intensive, but it may be relevant when a screening programme is started as part of operational research. It may be feasible to implement this type of data collection on a continual basis for certain risk groups, such as people seeking care in medical facilities;
- a register of all suspected cases of TB who undergo further diagnostic evaluation (if a register is used to collect individual-level information for all people who are screened, then this information can be included on it);
- a column in the laboratory register for noting whether the tested patient was identified through screening, and to which risk group the patient belongs;
- a column in the treatment register to note whether the patient was identified through screening, and to which risk group the patient belongs.

10.3   Programmatic evaluations

Based on the results of monitoring the indicators discussed above, a special assessment may be needed to explore, for example, the reasons for a low uptake of screening, an unexpectedly low proportion of people with suspected TB identified through screening, a low proportion of those with suspected TB having a diagnostic investigation, and a higher than expected number needed to screen. Additional quantitative and qualitative analyses may be needed to determine whether there are barriers to screening and to identify opportunities to improve the screening approach.

10.4   Monitoring time trends for reprioritization

A successful screening programme may lead to a diminishing yield over time, at least if the risk group is a fixed population. Over time, changes in the background burden of TB, as well as changes in the profile of TB patients in the community (for example, a trend towards fewer patients with symptomatic TB and fewer cases of smear-positive TB) can lead to a reduction in the yield from screening, an increase in the number needed to screen, a reduction in cost effectiveness, and a change in the ratio of benefits to harms. Trends in all of these indicators need to be monitored, and the prioritization of risk groups, choice of screening approach and screening interval should be regularly reassessed. Criteria for stopping screening should be established before a screening initiative is implemented.

10.5 Research

Standard monitoring and evaluation procedures may be complemented by operational research aimed at improving the performance of screening in the local setting as well as research aimed at improving the global evidence base on screening. Topics that may be explored include:
- assessing the accuracy and performance of different algorithms for screening and diagnosis;
- identifying operational challenges and solutions;
- identify the best ways to improve acceptability and minimize the harms of screening;
- establishing the effectiveness and cost effectiveness of screening in different risk groups and in different epidemiological situations

There is a need for more, larger and better randomized trials to assess the short-term and long-term effectiveness, and cost effectiveness, of screening. Implementing such studies requires careful planning and considerable resources.

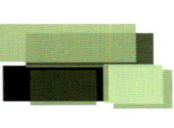

Annex I.

GRADE summary table: benefits of screening for tuberculosis (TB), all risk groups combined

(Details of the studies and full references are available in the supporting material on the Internet, see systematic review 1: the general benefits of TB screening[58].)

No. of studies	Quality assessment						Summary of findings				Quality	Importance
	Design	Limitations	Inconsistency	Indirectness	Imprecision	Other	No. of cases/population		Effect			
							Intervention	Control	Proportion of cases detected through screening of all cases			
1. Impact on case detection												
1.1 Cross-sectional studies assessing the proportion of cases detected through screening vs all notified cases												
Community-based screening, including screening in specific risk populations												
11[1]	Cross-sectional[2]	Serious[3]	Serious[4]	Not serious	Not serious	None	NA	NA	Range across studies: 6–86%		VERY LOW	IMPORTANT
Contact investigation												
5[5]	Cross-sectional[2]	Serious[3]	Not serious	Not serious	Not serious	None	NA	NA	Range across studies: 2–9% (19% in children aged <10, one study)		VERY LOW	

NA, not applicable; CI, confidence interval; RCT, randomized controlled trial; RR, relative risk.

---

[1] Meijer 1971, Meijer 1971b, Meijer 1971c, Meijer 1971d, Krivinka 1974, Aneja 1984, Harper 1996, Garcia 2000, Santha 2003, Gonzalez 2009, De Vries 2007.
[2] Cross-sectional study comparing the number of TB cases detected through screening with the total number of TB cases detected through screening and passive case-finding in the intervention area.
[3] None of the studies compared screening with an alternative intervention since in all settings screening was combined with passive case-detection. In all studies it is unknown whether cases detected through screening would have been detected through passive case-finding if screening had not been done. The study design does not allow for a direct assessment of the effect of screening on the detection of additional cases. The proportion of the population covered varied but was not consistently reported across the studies.
[4] There was large variation in the proportion of cases detected through screening; these variations were related to the differences across studies in the type and size of the target population, and differences in screening methods.
[5] Capewell 1984, Ormerod 1993, Jereb 1999, Lee 2008, Ottmani 2009.

Quality assessment							Summary of findings				Quality	Importance
No. of studies	Design	Limitations	Inconsistency	Indirectness	Imprecision	Other	No. of cases/population (No. cases/100 000)		Effect			
							Intervention	Control	Relative risk (95% CI)	Absolute (95% CI)		

1.2 Community-based randomized trials

Health-extension workers informed community about TB, identified people with TB symptoms and collected sputum samples at health posts once a month for 20 months; outcome: sputum smear-positive notification detection rate

| 1 (Datiko 2009) | RCT | Serious[6] | Only 1 trial | Serious[7] | Not serious | None | 230/178 138 (129/100 000) | 88/118 673 (74/100 000) | 1.55[8] | Case-detection rate: 53% higher in intervention clusters (40–65%)[9] | LOW | |

Community health promoters informed community about TB symptoms; sputum collection done during monthly outreach clinics in rural areas for 1 year; outcome: sputum smear-positive case notification rate

| 1 (Shargie 2006) | RCT | Serious[10] | Only 1 trial | Serious[16] | Serious[8] | None | 159/127 607 (125/100 000) | 221/225 284 (98/100 000) | 1.27 (0.81–1.72) | 27 more cases detected/100 000 population (from 19 fewer to 72 more) | VERY LOW | CRITICAL |

Repeated information campaigns about TB delivered to the community; decentralized sputum-collection points set up to provide easy access for community; sputum collected in health camps; intervention for 3 years; outcome: change in TB notification

| 1 (Ayles 2012) | RCT | Not serious | Only 1 trial | Serious[11] | Not serious | None | Cases at 0 years vs 3 years:875/946 (calculated ratio, 1.08) | Cases at 0 years vs 3 years:2024/2181 (calculated ratio, 1.08) | 1.0 | No difference in the change between intervention and control groups | MODERATE | |

[6] The method used to calculate the main outcome was unclear. The actual methods of screening and identifying people with TB symptoms was not clearly described. Randomization was described, but little baseline data are provided.
[7] Intervention assessed only in one setting.
[8] This is the crude ratio of case-notification rates; there were not enough data to calculate the confidence interval; adjusted for clustering
[9] The authors reported only the mean difference in case-detection rate, which conventionally is the ratio of case notification to the estimated incidence of TB, although the authors do not state exactly how it was calculated.
[10] The method for choosing which communities received the intervention was not described. Few baseline comparison data are given, but the map in the study suggests nonrandom selection, and that there were differences among intervention communities and control communities. The communities were contiguous so there could have been contamination.
[11] Intervention assessed in only one setting.

Quality assessment							Summary of findings					
							No. of cases/population (No. cases/100 000)		Effect			
No. of studies	Design	Limitations	Inconsistency	Indirectness	Imprecision	Other	Intervention	Control	Relative risk (95% CI)	Absolute (95% CI)	Quality	Importance
1.2 Community-based randomized trials												
Door-to-door screening for people with TB symptoms in poor urban areas												
1 (Miller 2010)	RCT	Not serious	Only 1 trial	Serious[11]	Serious[12]	None	N = 11 249; during intervention: 19 cases (notification rate, 934/100 000); 60 days after intervention: 32 cases: (516/100 000)	N = 12 304; during intervention: 16 cases (notification rate, 604/100 000); 60 days after intervention: 41cases (493/100 000)	During intervention: 1.55 (1.10–1.99); 60 days after intervention 1.05 (0.56–1.54	330/100 000 more cases (range, 60–598 more) during intervention; no difference 60 days after intervention	LOW	CRITICAL
Infants screened every 3 months through household visits; infants with suspected TB disease were investigated as inpatient in hospital												
1 (Moyo 2012)	RCT	Serious[13]	Only 1 trial	Serious[14]	Not serious	None	89/4109 person-years (2166/100 000)	36/4372 person-years (823/100 000)	2.6 (1.8–4.0)	1317 more cases detected/100 000 population per year (range, 659–2470 more)	LOW	

[12] The assessment of short-term impact was of borderline significance ; there was no significant impact after 60 days.

[13] The case definition includes the main criteria for determining a positive screening; possibility of overdiagnosis.

[14] Intervention assessed in only one setting; study looks at only young children.

2. Impact on time to diagnosis and disease severity at diagnosis

2.1 Studies of delay from reported onset of symptoms to start of treatment

No. of studies		Quality assessment						Summary of findings					
	Design	Limitations	Inconsistency	Indirectness	Imprecision	Other	Cases/pop., mean, or median		Effect		Quality	Importance
							Intervention	Control	RR (95% CI)	Absolute		

Studies of proportion of patients with delay >90 days; interventions used community outreach and sputum collection

| 1 (Shargie 2006a) | Cross-sectional | Serious[15] | Only 1 study | Serious[16] | Not serious | | 7/13 (54%) | 14/24 (58%) | 0.93 (0.50–1.69) | 4% fewer patients had delay >90 days in the screening group (from 50% fewer to 69% more) | VERY LOW | |

Studies of median delay, using door-to-door community-based screening

| 1 (Miller 2010) | RCT | Serious[12] | Only 1 study | Serious[16] | Not serious | | Median: 56 days | Median: 56 days | NA | No difference | LOW | |

Studies of mean time from birth to diagnosis in cohort of newborn children; door-to-door screening vs no screening

| 1 (Moyo 2012) | RCT | Serious[17] | Only 1 study | Serious[16] | Not serious | | Mean: 13.2 months | Mean: 16.6 months | NA | 3.4 months shorter time to diagnosis in screening group (from 0.3 months to 6.5 months shorter) | LOW | IMPORTANT |

Study of proportion of patients with delay >90 days; community outreach with sputum collection

| 1 (Shargie 2006b) | RCT | Serious | Only 1 study | Serious[16] | Not serious | | 65/159 (41%) | 139/221 (63%) | 0.65 (0.49–0.81) | 22/100 fewer had delay >90 days (12/100 to 32/100) | LOW | |

Proportion with cough lasting <3 weeks at time of diagnosis; community-based door-to-door screening

| 1 (Santha 2003)[18] | Cross-sectional | Serious | Only 1 study | Serious | Not serious | | Proportion: 37% | Proportion: 58% | 2.06 | 19/100 more with short duration in screened group | VERY LOW | |

---

[15] Self-reported onset of disease may not be reliable; recall bias may vary between screened cases and those passively detected. No study assessed change in delay after introduction of screening.
[16] Information from only one study.
[17] Most cases were diagnosed based on their symptoms not on microbiology; the case definition included the main criteria for a positive screening; overdiagnosis is likely to have occurred.
[18] The numerator and denominator are not available.

Quality assessment							Summary of findings				Quality	Importance
							Cases/pop., mean, or median		Effect			
No. of studies	Design	Limitations	Inconsistency	Indirectness	Imprecision	Other	Intervention	Control	RR (95% CI)	Absolute		
2.1 Studies of delay from reported onset of symptoms to start of treatment												IMPORTANT
Average delay; screening in prisons												
1 (Story 2008)[19]	Cross-sectional	Serious[20]	Only 1 study	Serious[21]	Serious[22]		NA	NA	3	NA	VERY LOW	
2.2 Studies of severity of disease at time of diagnosis												
Proportion of sputum smear-positive cases in people screened compared with passive case-finding												
13[23]	Cross-sectional	Not serious	Not serious	Serious[24]	Not serious		1093/2914 (38%)	3528/5373 (66%)	0.57 (0.54–0.60)	28/100 fewer people smear-positive in screened group (26/100 to 30/100 fewer)	VERY LOW	
Smear grade among sputum smear-positive cases; proportions reported as scanty, 2+ or 3+												
3[25]	Cross-sectional	Not serious	Not serious	Not serious	Not serious		147/345 (42%)	868/1308 (66%)	0.64 (0.56–0.73)	24/100 fewer reported 2+ or 3+ in screened group (18/100 to 29/100 fewer)	LOW	
Chest X-ray indicating severe disease												
3[26]	Cross-sectional	Serious	Minor	Serious	Minor		25/277 (22%)	659/4035 (68%)	0.41 (0.28–0.60)	40/100 fewer with severe X-ray findings in screened group (27/100 to 49/100 fewer)	VERY LOW	

[19] This study screened hard-to-reach groups, including homeless people, drug users, people in shelters and prisoners.
[20] Only a conference abstract is available, so design details cannot be assessed. The numerator and denominator are not available.
[21] The study did not report results separately for different subgroups; data from only one study.
[22] Absolute numbers are not available.
[23] Meijer 1971a, Meijer 1971b, Meijer 1971c, Meijer 1971d, Krivinka 1974, Ross 1977, Capewell 1986, LeBue 2004, den Boon 2008, , Shetty 2008, Story 2008, Eang 2012, Moyo 2012.
[24] The method of diagnosis was not necessarily the same in groups that were screened and groups that were not screened.
[25] Shetty 1999, den Boon 2008, Eang 2012.
[26] Ross 1977, Wang 2000, LeBue 2004.

	Quality assessment						Summary of findings					
							No. of cases/population (No. cases/100 000 or %)		Effect			
No. of studies	Design	Limitations	Inconsistency	Indirectness	Imprecision	Other	Intervention	Control	Relative risk (95% CI)	Absolute	Quality	Importance

3. Impact on treatment outcomes

Treatment success rate; compared treatment outcomes in cohorts identified by screening with cohorts identified by passive case-finding

| 6[27] | Cohort | Serious[28] | No | No | Serious[29] | No | 1202/1496 (80%) | 4827/6199 (78%) | Pooled RR: 1.0 (0.98–1.02) | Same proportion successfully treated | VERY LOW | CRITICAL |

Death rate only (TB-specific mortality); population assessed was miners

| 1 (Churchyard 2000) | Cohort | No | No | No | Serious[30] | No | 12/1225 (1.0%) | 69/1011 (6.8%) | Adjusted RR: 5.6 (2.6–12.2) | 5.5 fewer deaths/100 treated (4.2 to 6.3 fewer/100 treated) | VERY LOW | CRITICAL |

[27] Cassels 1982, Harper 1996, Santha 2003, den Boon 2008, Ayles 2012. Eang 2012.
[28] Findings were not controlled for disease severity at time of diagnosis and other patient-related factors.
[29] None of the studies compared change in treatment success rate after screening was introduced.
[30] Information from only one study.

| | | Quality assessment | | | | | Summary of findings | | | | | |
| | | | | | | | No. of cases/population | | | Effect | | |
No. of studies	Design	Limitations	Inconsistency	Indirectness	Imprecision	Other	Intervention	Control	RR (95% CI)	Absolute	Quality	Importance

4. Impact on TB epidemiology in the community

Continual mandatory screening and treatment of active and latent TB among people using homeless shelters in a setting with a moderate burden; compared incidence after intervention with baseline incidence in intervention district; study lasted for 10 years

1 (Rendelman 1999)	Secular trend; before vs after	Serious[31]	Only 1 study	Serious[32]	Not serious	None	5 /17241 (29/100 000)	39/17180 (227/100 00 0)	0.13 (0.05– 0.32)	34 fewer cases, or 198/100 000 in intervention district 10 years after screening was introduced (from 154 to 215/100 000)	VERY LOW	CRITICAL

One-time household screening in randomly selected clusters in high-burden setting; compared smear-positive notification rate in intervention clusters with national rate 2 years after screening

1 (Okada 2012)	Cohort study	Serious[31]	Only 1 study	Serious[32]	Not serious	None	34 (154/100 000)	89.5 (404/100 00 0)	0.38 (0.27– 0.52)	250 fewer smear-positive cases/ 100 000 population 2 years after one-off screening	VERY LOW	

Screening of household TB contacts; included providing chemoprophylaxis for those with likely latent infection; high-burden setting; compared TB notification in intervention and control areas; study lasted for 5 years

1 (Cavalcante 2010)	Cluster RCT	Not serious	Only 1 study	Serious[32]	Serious[33]	None	339 to 305/100 000 (10% decrease)[34]	340 to 358/100 000 (5% increase)[32]	NA	15% difference in change of incidence (P for difference, 0.04)	LOW	

---

[31] No control group

[32] Only one setting

[33] Borderline statistical significance

[34] The absolute number of cases by year was not reported.

Quality assessment							Summary of findings					
							No. of cases/population		Effect			
No. of studies	Design	Limitations	Inconsistency	Indirectness	Imprecision	Other	Intervention	Control	RR (95% CI)	Absolute	Quality	Import-ance
Community screening every 6 months with mobile van or door-to-door visits *vs* baseline preintervention; high-burden setting; compared TB prevalence before and after intervention; study lasted for 3 years												
1 (Corbett 2010)	Cluster RCT	Serious[35]	Only 1 study	Serious[32]	Not serious		41/11 081 (370/100 000)	66/10 153 (650/100 000)	Adjusted RR: 0.59 (0.40–0.89)	280 fewer prevalent cases/100 000 after 3 years (from 71 to 390/100 000 fewer)	LOW	
Cluster randomized trial of community outreach and sputum collection *vs* household intervention (3 visits per household, including screening of household contacts)[36] *vs* neither intervention; evaluated prevalence of active TB and infection incidence; study lasted 3 years												
1 (Ayles 2012) a. Community outreach b. Household intervention	Cluster RCT	Not serious	Only 1 study	Serious[37]	a. Not serious b. Serious[38]		a. TB prevalence: 927/100 000; infection incidence: 1.41% b. TB prevalence: 746/100 000; infection incidence: 0.87%	a. TB prevalence: 711/100 000; infection incidence: 1.05% b. TB prevalence: 883/100 000; infection incidence: 1.71%	a. Adjusted RR TB: 1.11 (0.87–1.42); adjusted RR infection: 1.36 (0.59–3.14) b. Adjusted RR TB: 0.78 (0.61–1.00); adjusted RR infection: 0.45 (0.20–1.05)	a. 216/100 000 higher prevalence in intervention areas (range, from 92 less to 299 more); 3.6/1000 higher infection incidence in intervention arm (range, 4.3 to 22/1000) b. 194 fewer prevalent TB cases/100 000 population in intervention areas; 0.9 fewer infections/100 population in intervention areas	a. MODERATE b. LOW	CRITICAL

35 There was no control area without an intervention; there were only two different interventions; difficult to control for secular trend.

36 The study also included an arm that had enhanced case-finding, but which did not include actual screening; those results are not reported here.

37 Data from only one study in a specific epidemiological situation; household intervention included a screening element but also other interactions, including treatment of latent TB and HIV counselling, testing and management for household members.

38 For the household-intervention arm, the impact on the prevalence of active TB was borderline statistically significant; the impact on prevalence of TB infection was not statistically significant.

Quality assessment							Summary of findings					Import-ance
No. of studies	Design	Limitations	Inconsistency	Indirectness	Imprecision	Other	No. of cases/population		Effect		Quality	
							Intervention	Control	RR (95% CI)	Absolute		
Impact only within the risk group; decline in incidence												CRITICAL
1 (De Vries 2007)	Secular trend	Serious[39]	Only 1 study	Serious[40]	Not serious		11/4500 (244/100 000)	24/4500 (553/100 000)	0.46 (0.22–0.93)	309/100 000 fewer incident cases after intervention (from 34 to 431 fewer)	VERY LOW	
1 study[41] (Yanjindulam 2012)	Longitu dinal surveill ance	Serious[42]	Only 1 study	Serious[43]	Serious[44]		900/100 000 in prison population in 2010	2500/100 000 in prison population in 2001	0.36	1600/100 000 notified cases fewer after 10 years; stable national notification trend	VERY LOW	

---

[39] This study had no control group, and only compared changes before the intervention versus after the intervention within the risk group.

[40] Data from only one study in one setting.

[41] Study assessed the introduction of systematic screening during both detention and at time of conviction, combined with improved TB management and improved living conditions in the prisons, between 2001 and 2010; included 23 prisons and 16 detention centres with a total of about 6000 prisoners. Trend in TB notification within prisons was compared with national trend.

[42] There was no control group; study compared only trends in prisons before and after the intervention with national trends during the same period.

[43] Data from only one study in one setting. It is not possible to separate the impact of screening from the impact of improved living conditions and improved TB treatment.

[44] Data do not allow for calculation of statistical uncertainty.

GRADE summary tables: sensitivity and specificity of screening tools for tuberculosis (TB)

Table 1. **What is the accuracy of chest X-rays in identifying active TB during screening in the general population?**

Index test: chest X-ray – any abnormality | Reference test: sputum culture or sputum-smear microscopy, or both

Place where test is offered: triage

Outcomes	No. of studies (No. of participants)	Study design	Factors that may decrease the quality of evidence					Quality of evidence	Effect per 100 000 with 98% sensitivity (95–100%)[f] and 75% specificity (72–79%)
			Limitations in study design[a]	Indirectness[b]	Inconsistency[c]	Imprecision[d]	Publication bias[e]		
True positives (active TB)	3 (72 065)	Cross-sectional	Serious	None	None	None	NA	Moderate	At prevalence 0.25%: 245 (238–250) At prevalence 1%: 980 (950–100)
False negatives (incorrectly classified as no active TB)									At prevalence 0.25%: 5 (0–13) At prevalence 1%: 20 (0–50)
True negatives (no active TB)	3 (72 065)	Cross-sectional	Serious	None	None	None	NA	Moderate	At prevalence 0.25%: 74 813 (71 820–78 803) At prevalence 1%: 74 250 (72 280–78 210)
False positives (incorrectly classified as active TB)									At prevalence 0.25%: 24 938 (20 948–27 930) At prevalence 1%: 24 750 (20 790–27 720)

Studies included: den Boon, 2006; Ministry of Health, Myanmar, 2012; Van 't Hoog, 2012. (Details of the studies are available in the supporting material on the Internet at www.who.int/tb/tbscreening.)

NA, not applicable.

[a] Limitations in study design (see QUADAS-2):[47] there is a high risk of selection bias in one study (den Boon, 2006). In all studies, less than half of the participants received the reference standard (range, 23–45%); accuracy was calculated under the assumption that those who did not receive the reference standard were culture-negative or smear-negative, or both – that is, they did not have active TB.

[b] Indirectness (see QUADAS-2):[47] there is some concern about the applicability of the reference standard in two studies – no downgrading.

[c] Inconsistency: there were homogenous results for sensitivity and specificity (based on visual inspection of the confidence intervals).

[d] Imprecision: estimates for sensitivity and specificity are precise.

[e] Publication bias: this concern is not applicable for these studies; the evidence base for publication bias in studies assessing the accuracy of diagnostic tests is limited.

[f] Values in parentheses are 95% confidence intervals.

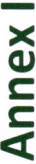

Table 2. **What is the accuracy of chest x-rays in identifying active TB during screening in the general population?**

Index test: chest X-ray – TB-related abnormalities | Reference test: sputum culture or sputum-smear microscopy, or both

Place where test is offered: triage

Test–treatment pathway: positive chest X-ray => confirmatory test (mycobacterial culture or Xpert MTB/RIF) => anti-TB chemotherapy (6–9 months of antibiotics)

Outcomes	No. of studies (No. of participants)	Study design	Factors that may decrease the quality of evidence					Quality of evidence	Effect per 100 000 with 87% sensitivity (79–95%)[f] and 89% specificity (87–92%)
			Limitations in study design[a]	Indirectness[b]	Inconsistency[c]	Imprecision[d]	Publication bias[e]		
True positives (active TB)	5 (163 646)	Cross-sectional	Very serious	None	None	None	NA	Low	At prevalence 0.25%: 218 (198–238) / At prevalence 1%: 870 (790–950)
False negatives (incorrectly classified as no active TB)									At prevalence 0.25%: 33 (13–53) / At prevalence 1%: 130 (50–210)
True negatives (no active TB)	5 (163 646)	Cross-sectional	Very serious	None	None	None	NA	Low	At prevalence 0.25%: 88 778 (86 783–91 770) / At prevalence 1%: 88 110 (86 130–91 080)
False positives (incorrectly classified as active TB)									At prevalence 0.25%: 10 973 (7 980–12 968) / At prevalence 1%: 10 890 (7 920–12 870)

Studies included: Ministry of Health, Cambodia, 2005; den Boon, 2006; Hoa, 2012; Ministry of Health, Myanmar, 2012; Van 't Hoog, 2012. (Details of the studies are available in the supporting material on the Internet at www.who.int/tb/tbscreening.)

NA, not applicable.

[a] Limitations in study design (see QUADAS-2):[47] there is a high risk of selection bias in one study (den Boon, 2006); in three studies the risk of bias is unclear for the reference standard. In all studies, less than half of the participants received the reference standard (range, 8–45%); accuracy was calculated under the assumption that those who did not receive the reference standard were culture-negative or smear-negative, or both – that is, they did not have active TB.

[b] Indirectness (see QUADAS-2):[47] there is concern about the applicability of the reference standard in two studies – no downgrading.

[c] Inconsistency: there was moderate heterogeneity for sensitivity (based on visual inspection of the confidence intervals); there was little heterogeneity for specificity – no downgrading.

[d] Imprecision: estimates for sensitivity and specificity are imprecise.

[e] Publication bias: this concern is not applicable for these studies; the evidence base for publication bias in studies assessing the accuracy of diagnostic tests is limited.

[f] Values in parentheses are 95% confidence intervals.

Table 3. **What is the accuracy of screening for cough to identify active TB during screening in the general population?**

Index test: prolonged cough | Reference test: sputum culture or sputum-smear microscopy, or both

Place where test is offered: triage

Test-treatment pathway: positive for cough => confirmatory test (mycobacterial culture or Xpert MTB/RIF) => anti-TB chemotherapy (6–9 months of antibiotics)

Outcomes	No. of studies (No. of participants)	Study design	Factors that may decrease the quality of evidence					Quality of evidence	Effect per 100 000 with 35% sensitivity (24–46%)[f] and 95% specificity (93–97%)
			Limitations in study design[a]	Indirectness[b]	Inconsistency[c]	Imprecision[d]	Publication bias[e]		
True positives (active TB)	8 (223 402)	Cross-sectional	Very serious	None	None	Serious	NA	Very low	At prevalence 0.25%: 88 (60–115) At prevalence 1%: 350 (240–460)
False negatives (incorrectly classified as no active TB)									At prevalence 0.25%: 163 (135–190) At prevalence 1%: 650 (540–760)
True negatives (no active TB)	8 (223 402)	Cross-sectional	Very serious	None	None	None	NA	Low	At prevalence 0.25%: 94 763 (92 768–96 758) At prevalence 1%: 94 050 (92 070–96 030)
False positives (incorrectly classified as active TB)									At prevalence 0.25%: 4988 (2993–6983) At prevalence 1%: 4950 (2970–6930)

Studies included: Datta, 2001; Ministry of Health, Cambodia, 2005; den Boon, 2006; Ayles, 2009; Corbett, 2010; Hoa, 2012; Ministry of Health, Myanmar 2012; Van 't Hoog, 2012. (Details of the studies are available in the supporting material on the Internet at www.who.int/tb/tbscreening.)

NA, not applicable.

[a] Limitations in study design (see QUADAS-2):[47] there is a high risk of selection bias in one study (den Boon, 2006); in one study the risk of bias is unclear for the index test; and in three studies the risk of bias is unclear for the reference standard. In six of the eight studies, less than half of the participants received the reference standard (range, 8–45%); accuracy was calculated under the assumption that those who did not receive the reference standard were culture-negative or smear-negative, or both – that is they did not have active TB.

[b] Indirectness (see QUADAS-2):[47] there is concern about the applicability of the reference standard in three studies – no downgrading.

[c] Inconsistency: there was moderate heterogeneity for sensitivity (based on visual inspection the confidence intervals); there was little heterogeneity for specificity – no downgrading.

[d] Imprecision: the estimates for sensitivity were imprecise; there were precise estimates for specificity.

[e] Publication bias: this concern is not applicable for these studies; the evidence base for publication bias in studies assessing the accuracy of diagnostic tests is limited.

[f] Values in parentheses are 95% confidence intervals.

Table 4. **What is the accuracy of screening for cough to identify active TB during screening in the general population?**

Index test: prolonged cough | Reference test: sputum-smear microscopy

Place where test is offered: triage

Test–treatment pathway: positive cough positive => confirmatory test (mycobacterial culture or Xpert MTB/RIF) => anti-TB chemotherapy (6–9 months of antibiotics)

Outcomes	No. of studies (No. of participants)	Study design	Factors that may decrease the quality of evidence					Quality of evidence	Effect per 100 000 with 56% sensitivity (42–74%)[f] and 92% specificity (87–98%)
			Limitations in study design[a]	Indirectness[b]	Inconsistency[c]	Imprecision[d]	Publication bias[e]		
True positives (active TB)	4 (95 188)	Cross-sectional	Very serious	None	None	Serious	NA	Very low	At prevalence 0.25%: 140 (105–185) / At prevalence 1%: 560 (420–740)
False negatives (incorrectly classified as no active TB)									At prevalence 0.25%: 110 (65–145) / At prevalence 1%: 440 (260–580)
True negatives (no active TB)	4 (95 188)	Cross-sectional	Very serious	None	None	Serious	NA	Very low	At prevalence 0.25%: 91 770 (86 783–97 755) / At prevalence 1%: 91 080 (86 130–97 020)
False positives (incorrectly classified as active TB)									At prevalence 0.25%: 7 980 (1 995–12 968) / At prevalence 1%: 7 920 (1 980–12 870)

Studies included: Ministry of Health, Cambodia, 2005; den Boon, 2006; Ministry of Health, Myanmar, 2012; Van 't Hoog, 2012. (Details of the studies are available in the supporting material on the Internet at www.who.int/tb/tbscreening.)

NA, not applicable.

[a] Limitations in study design (see QUADAS-2):[47] there is a high risk of selection bias in one study (den Boon, 2006); in two studies the risk of bias is unclear for the reference standard. In all studies, less than half of the participants received the reference standard (range, 15–45%); accuracy was calculated under the assumption that those who did not receive the reference standard were culture-negative or smear-negative, or both – that is, they did not have active TB.

[b] Indirectness (see QUADAS-2):[47] there are no major concerns about applicability.

[c] Inconsistency: there was moderate heterogeneity for sensitivity (based on visual inspection of the confidence intervals); there was little heterogeneity for specificity – no downgrading.

[d] Imprecision: the estimates for sensitivity and specificity were imprecise (with wide confidence intervals for false-negatives and false-positives).

[e] Publication bias: this concern is not applicable for these studies; the evidence base for publication bias in studies assessing the accuracy of diagnostic tests is limited

[f] Values in parentheses are 95% confidence intervals.

Table 5. **What is the accuracy of screening for cough to identify active TB during screening in the general population?**

Index test: any cough| Reference test: sputum culture or sputum-smear microscopy, or both

Place where test is offered: triage

Test-treatment pathway: positive cough => confirmatory test (mycobacterial culture or Xpert MTB/RIF) => anti-TB chemotherapy (6–9 months of antibiotics)

| Outcomes | No. of studies (No. of participants) | Study design | Factors that may decrease the quality of evidence | | | | | Quality of evidence | Effect per 100 000 with 56% sensitivity (40–74%)[f] and 80% specificity (69–90%) |
			Limitations in study design[a]	Indirect-ness[b]	Incons-istency[c]	Imprec-ision[d]	Publication bias[e]		
True positives (active TB)	7 (131 052)	Cross-sectional	Serious	None	None	Serious	NA	Low	At prevalence 0.25%: 140 (100–185) At prevalence 1%: 560 (400–470)
False negatives (incorrectly classified as no active TB)									At prevalence 0.25%: 110 (65–150) At prevalence 1%: 440 (260–600)
True negatives (no active TB)	7 (131 052)	Cross-sectional	Serious	None	None	Serious	NA	Low	At prevalence 0.25%: 79 800 (68 828–89 775) At prevalence 1%: 79 200 (68 310–89 100)
False positives (incorrectly classified as active TB)									At prevalence 0.25%: 19 800 (9 975–30 923) At prevalence 1%: 7 920 (9 900–30 690)

Studies included: Ministry of Health, Cambodia, 2005; Wood, 2006; Sebhatu, 2007; Ayles, 2009; Corbett, 2010; Ministry of Health, Myanmar, 2012; Van 't Hoog, 2012. (Details of the studies are available in the supporting material on the Internet at www.who.int/tb/tbscreening.)

NA, not applicable.

[a] Limitations in study design (see QUADAS-2):[47] in three of the seven studies less than half of the participants received the reference standard (range, 15–32%); accuracy was calculated under the assumption that those who did not receive the reference standard were culture-negative or smear-negative, or both – that is, they did not have active TB.

[b] Indirectness (see QUADAS-2):[47] there are no major concerns about applicability.

[c] Inconsistency: there was moderate heterogeneity for sensitivity and specificity (based on visual inspection of the confidence intervals) – no downgrading.

[d] Imprecision: the estimates for sensitivity and specificity were imprecise (with wide confidence intervals for false-negatives and false-positives).

[e] Publication bias: this concern is not applicable for these studies; the evidence base for publication bias in studies assessing the accuracy of diagnostic tests is limited.

[f] Values in parentheses are 95% confidence intervals.

Table 6. **What is the accuracy of screening for any symptom to identify active TB during screening in a general population with a low prevalence of HIV?**

Index test: any symptom| Reference test: sputum culture or sputum-smear microscopy, or both

Place where test is offered: triage

Test–treatment pathway: positive symptom => confirmatory test (mycobacterial culture or Xpert MTB/RIF) => anti-TB chemotherapy (6–9 months of antibiotics)

Outcomes	No. of studies (No. of participants)	Study design	Factors that may decrease the quality of evidence					Quality of evidence	Effect per 100 000 with 70% sensitivity (58–82%)[f] and 61% specificity (35–87%)
			Limitations in study design[a]	Indirectness[b]	Inconsistency[c]	Imprecision[d]	Publication bias[e]		
True positives (active TB)	4 (178 376)	Cross-sectional	Very serious	None	None	Serious	NA	Very low	At prevalence 0.25%: 175 (145–205) At prevalence 1%: 700 (580–820)
False negatives (incorrectly classified as no active TB)									At prevalence 0.25%: 75 (45–105) At prevalence 1%: 300 (180–420)
True negatives (no active TB)	4 (178 376)	Cross-sectional	Very serious	None	None	Serious	NA	Very low	At prevalence 0.25%: 60 848 (34 913–86 783) At prevalence 1%: 60 390 (34 650–86 130)
False positives (incorrectly classified as active TB)									At prevalence 0.25%: 38 903 (12 968–64 838) At prevalence 1%: 38 610 (12 870–64 350)

Studies included: Datta, 2001; Gopi, 2003; Ministry of Health, Cambodia, 2005; Ministry of Health, Myanmar, 2012. (Details of the studies are available in the supporting material on the Internet at www.who.int/tb/tbscreening.)

NA, not applicable.

[a] Limitations in study design (see QUADAS-2):[47] in all studies less than 25% of the participants received the reference standard (range, 11–23%); accuracy was calculated under the assumption that those who did not receive the reference standard were culture-negative or smear-negative, or both – that is, they did not have active TB.

[b] Indirectness (see QUADAS-2):[47] there were no major concerns about .applicability.

[c] Inconsistency: there is moderate heterogeneity for sensitivity and specificity (based on visual inspection of the confidence intervals) – no downgrading.

[d] Imprecision: the estimates for sensitivity and specificity were imprecise (with wide confidence intervals for false-negatives and false-positives).

[e] Publication bias: this concern is not applicable for these studies; the evidence base for publication bias in studies assessing the accuracy of diagnostic tests is limited.

[f] Values in parentheses are 95% confidence intervals.

Table 7. **What is the accuracy of screening for any symptom to identify active TB during screening in a general population with a high prevalence of HIV?**

Index test: any symptom | Reference test: sputum culture or sputum-smear microscopy, or both

Place where the test is offered: triage

Test–treatment pathway: positive symptom => confirmatory test (mycobacterial culture or Xpert MTB/RIF) => anti-TB chemotherapy (6–9 months of antibiotics)

Outcomes	No. of studies (No. of participants)	Study design	Factors that may decrease the quality of evidence					Quality of evidence	Effect per 100 000 with 84% sensitivity (77–93%)[f] and 74% specificity (53–95%)
			Limitations in study design[a]	Indirectness[b]	Inconsistency[c]	Imprecision[d]	Publication bias[e]		
True positives (active TB)	4 (40 100)	Cross-sectional	Serious	None	None	Serious	NA	Low	At prevalence 0.25%: 210 (193–233) At prevalence 1%: 840 (770–930)
False negatives (incorrectly classified as no active TB)	(40 100)	Cross-sectional	Serious	None	None	Serious	NA	Low	At prevalence 0.25%: 40 (18–58) At prevalence 1%: 160 (70–230)
True negatives (no active TB)	4 (40 100)	Cross-sectional	Serious	None	None	Very serious	NA	Very low	At prevalence 0.25%: 73 815 (52 868–94 763) At prevalence 1%: 73 260 (52 470–94 050)
False positives (incorrectly classified as active TB)	(40 100)	Cross-sectional	Serious	None	None	Very serious	NA	Very low	At prevalence 0.25%: 25 935 (4 988–46 883) At prevalence 1%: 25 740 (4 950–46 530)

Studies included: den Boon, 2006; Ayles, 2009; Corbett, 2010; Van 't Hoog, 2012. (Details of the studies are available in the supporting material on the Internet at www.who.int/tb/tbscreening.)

NA, not applicable.

[a] Limitations in study design (see QUADAS-2).[47] in two of the four studies less than half of the participants received the reference standard (range, 32–44%); accuracy was calculated under the assumption that those who did not receive the reference standard were culture-negative or smear-negative, or both – that is, they did not have active TB.

[b] Indirectness (see QUADAS-2):[47] there are no major concerns about applicability.

[c] Inconsistency: there were homogenous results for sensitivity, and considerable heterogeneity for specificity (based on visual inspection of the confidence intervals) – no downgrading.

[d] Imprecision: the estimates for sensitivity and specificity were imprecise (with wide confidence intervals for false-negatives and false-positives).

[e] Publication bias: this concern is not applicable for these studies; the evidence base for publication bias in studies assessing the accuracy of diagnostic tests is limited.

[f] Values in parentheses are 95% confidence intervals.

Table 8. **What is the accuracy of screening for any symptom to identify active TB during screening in the general population?**

Index test: any symptom| Reference test: sputum culture or sputum-smear microscopy, or both

Place where test is offered: triage

Test–treatment pathway: positive symptom => confirmatory test (mycobacterial culture or Xpert MTB/RIF) => anti-TB chemotherapy (6–9 months of antibiotics)

Outcomes	No. of studies (No. of participants)	Study design	Factors that may decrease the quality of evidence					Quality of evidence	Effect per 100 000 with 77% sensitivity (68–86%)[f] and 68% specificity (50–85%)
			Limitations in study design[a]	Indirectness[b]	Inconsistency[c]	Imprecision[d]	Publication bias[e]		
True positives (active TB)	8 (218 476)	Cross-sectional	Very serious	None	None	Serious	NA	Very low	At prevalence 0.25%: 193 (170–215) At prevalence 1%: 770 (680–860)
False negatives (incorrectly classified as no active TB)									At prevalence 0.25%: 58 (35–80) At prevalence 1%: 230 (140–320)
True negatives (no active TB)	8 (218 476)	Cross-sectional	Very serious	None	None	Very serious	NA	Very low	At prevalence 0.25%: 67 830 (49 875–84 788) At prevalence 1%: 67 320 49 500–84 150)
False positives (incorrectly classified as active TB)									At prevalence 0.25%: 31 920 (14 963–49 875) At prevalence 1%: 31 680 (14 850–49 500)

Studies included: Datta, 2001; Gopi, 2003; Ministry of Health, Cambodia, 2005; den Boon, 2006; Ayles, 2009; Corbett, 2010; Ministry of Health, Myanmar, 2012; Van 't Hoog, 2012. (Details of the studies are available in the supporting material on the Internet at www.who.int/tb/tbscreening.)

NA, not applicable.

[a] Limitations in study design (see QUADAS-2):[47] there is a high risk of selection bias in one study (den Boon, 2006); in two studies the risk of bias is unclear for the reference standard. In six of the eight studies less than half of the participants received the reference standard (range, 11–44%); accuracy was calculated under the assumption that those who did not receive the reference standard were culture-negative or smear-negative, or both – that is, they did not have active TB.

[b] Indirectness (see QUADAS-2):[47] there are no major concerns about applicability. [c] Inconsistency: there was moderate heterogeneity for sensitivity, and considerable heterogeneity for specificity (based on visual inspection of the confidence intervals) – no downgrading.

[d] Imprecision: the estimates for sensitivity and specificity were imprecise (with wide confidence intervals for false-negatives and false-positives).

[e] Publication bias: this concern is not applicable for these studies; the evidence base for publication bias in studies assessing the accuracy of diagnostic tests is limited.

[f] Values in parentheses are 95% confidence intervals.

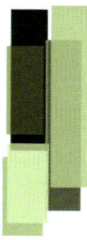

Annex III.

Flow charts of algorithms for screening and diagnosing tuberculosis (TB) in adults, with modelled yields and predictive values

Screening algorithms options are presented in section9. Each algorithm for adults includes options for the initial diagnostic testing of people whose screening test is positive: either sputum-smear microscopy (conventional light microscopy used to examine direct smears stained with Ziehl–Neelsen, with or without specific sputum-processing methods, or fluorescence microscopy including microscopy with light-emitting diodes) or a rapid molecular test that has been demonstrated to have high accuracy, such as the Xpert MTB/RIF test (Cepheid, Sunnyvale, CA) (or any rapid test recommended by WHO in the future that has the same or better accuracy than the Xpert MTB/RIF).

Positive or negative diagnostic results may require a repeat test or further diagnostic evaluation using culture, drug-susceptibility testing, clinical assessment, or some combination of these. In these algorithms, culture is not considered for use as an initial diagnostic test because it requires a much longer wait for results (2–6 weeks) than both nucleic acid amplification tests (such as the Xpert MTB/RIF test) and sputum-smear microscopy, both of which can provide final test results in less than 1 day.

The choice of algorithm depends on the risk group being evaluated, the prevalence of TB, the availability of resources and the feasibility (see Sections 8 and 9).

For each algorithm, the following estimates are provided for different prevalences of TB (0.5%, 1% and 2%) in the screened population:
- negative predictive values of the screening test;
- pretest probability for the initial diagnostic test;
- positive predictive value and negative predictive value of the initial diagnostic test among people whose screening test is positive;

- proportion of true cases detected by the algorithm using outcomes from only the initial diagnostic test;
- proportion of those with a negative result on the initial diagnostic test that is assumed to undergo further diagnosis with chest X-ray (if not already done) and clinical assessment (see support material at www.who.int/tb/tbscreening);
- proportion of true cases detected by the algorithm using the results of the initial diagnostic test plus clinical diagnosis in the proportion of those with a negative result on the diagnostic test that is assumed to undergo clinical diagnosis;
- positive predictive value when using the combination of the initial diagnostic test and clinical diagnosis.

Definitions of estimates used to evaluate the algorithms

Positive predictive value (PPV): the likelihood that a person diagnosed with TB has true culture-positive TB (also the proportion of all detected cases that are true culture-positive TB cases)

Negative predictive value (NPV): the likelihood that a person who is not diagnosed with TB does not have culture-positive TB (1 − NPV = the probability that a person not diagnosed with TB actually has culture-positive TB)

Pretest probability (PTP): the prevalence of culture-positive TB among persons eligible for a test (for a second test in an algorithm this equals the PPV of the previous test); the pretest probability increases with each screening step

Algorithm 1a (chest X-ray and Xpert MTB/RIF not available)

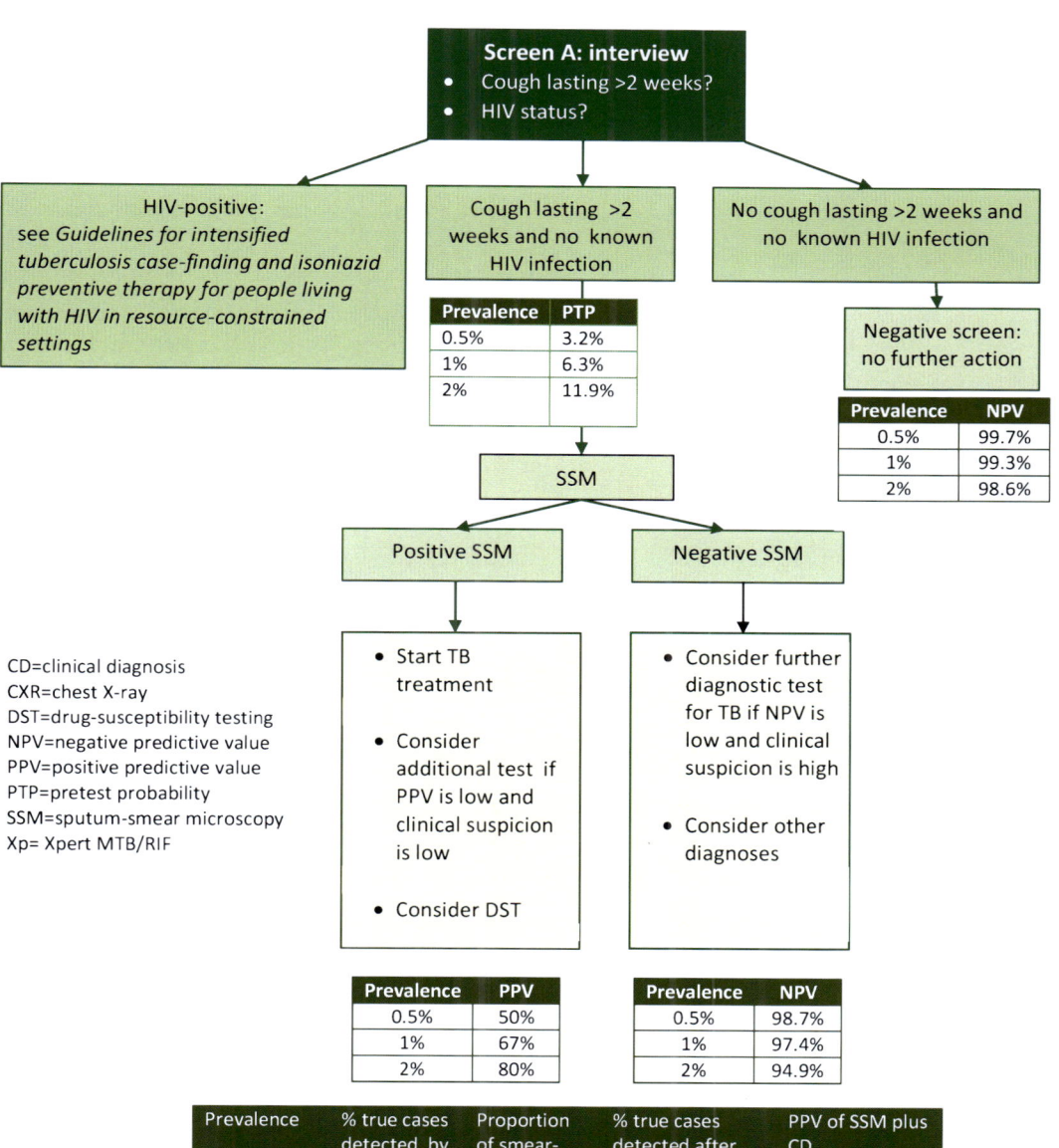

Screen A: interview
- Cough lasting >2 weeks?
- HIV status?

HIV-positive:
see *Guidelines for intensified tuberculosis case-finding and isoniazid preventive therapy for people living with HIV in resource-constrained settings*

Cough lasting >2 weeks and no known HIV infection

Prevalence	PTP
0.5%	3.2%
1%	6.3%
2%	11.9%

No cough lasting >2 weeks and no known HIV infection

Negative screen: no further action

Prevalence	NPV
0.5%	99.7%
1%	99.3%
2%	98.6%

SSM

Positive SSM

Negative SSM

CD=clinical diagnosis
CXR=chest X-ray
DST=drug-susceptibility testing
NPV=negative predictive value
PPV=positive predictive value
PTP=pretest probability
SSM=sputum-smear microscopy
Xp= Xpert MTB/RIF

- Start TB treatment

- Consider additional test if PPV is low and clinical suspicion is low

- Consider DST

- Consider further diagnostic test for TB if NPV is low and clinical suspicion is high

- Consider other diagnoses

Prevalence	PPV
0.5%	50%
1%	67%
2%	80%

Prevalence	NPV
0.5%	98.7%
1%	97.4%
2%	94.9%

Prevalence	% true cases detected by SSM only	Proportion of smear-negative that go to CD	% true cases detected after SSM plus CD	PPV of SSM plus CD
0.5%	21%	20%	22%	40%
1%	21%	30%	22%	53%
2%	21%	60%	23%	62%

Algorithm 1b (chest X-ray not available, Xpert MTB/RIF available)

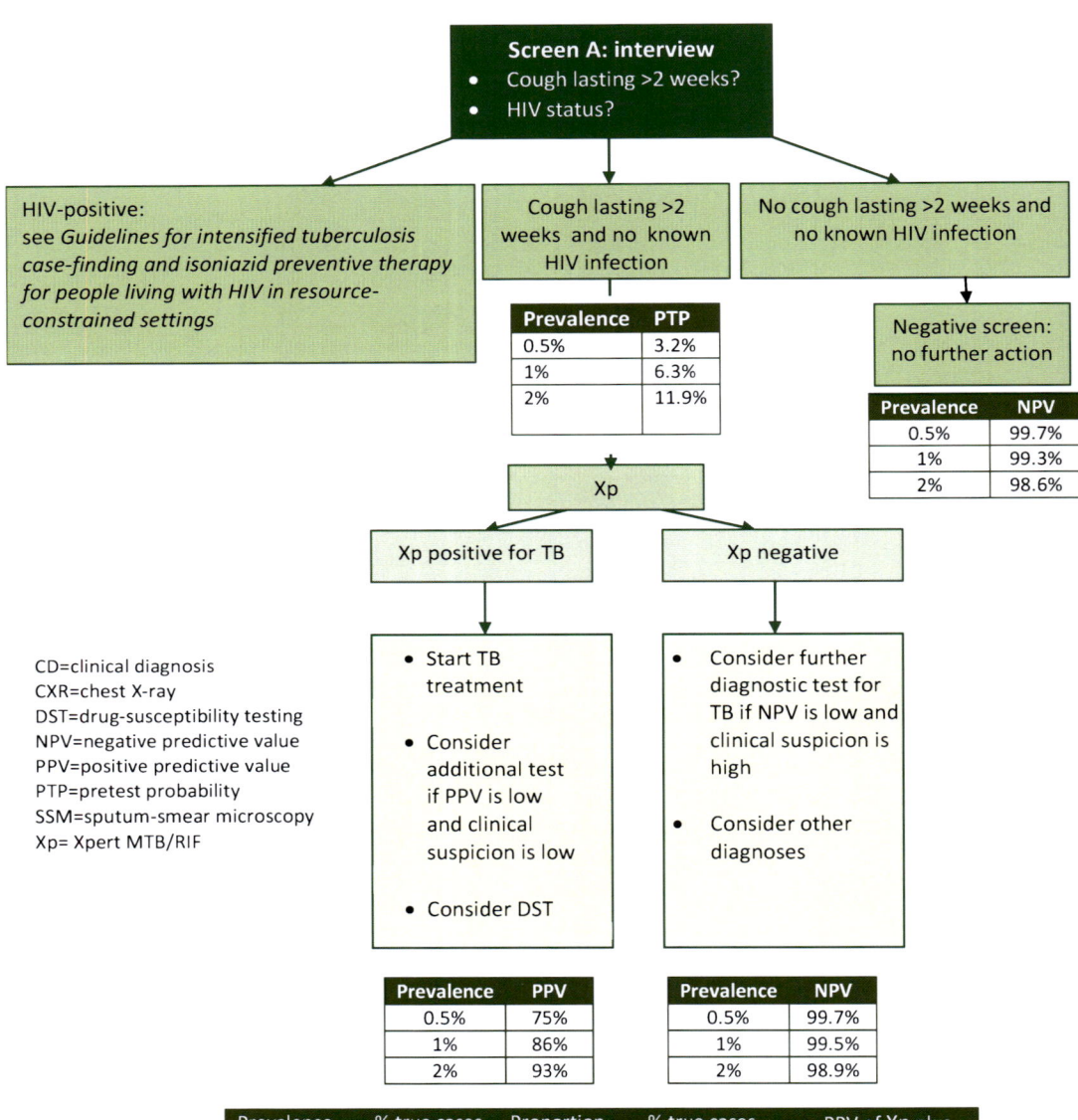

Screen A: interview
- Cough lasting >2 weeks?
- HIV status?

HIV-positive:
see *Guidelines for intensified tuberculosis case-finding and isoniazid preventive therapy for people living with HIV in resource-constrained settings*

Cough lasting >2 weeks and no known HIV infection

No cough lasting >2 weeks and no known HIV infection

Prevalence	PTP
0.5%	3.2%
1%	6.3%
2%	11.9%

Negative screen: no further action

Prevalence	NPV
0.5%	99.7%
1%	99.3%
2%	98.6%

Xp

Xp positive for TB

Xp negative

- Start TB treatment
- Consider additional test if PPV is low and clinical suspicion is low
- Consider DST

- Consider further diagnostic test for TB if NPV is low and clinical suspicion is high
- Consider other diagnoses

CD=clinical diagnosis
CXR=chest X-ray
DST=drug-susceptibility testing
NPV=negative predictive value
PPV=positive predictive value
PTP=pretest probability
SSM=sputum-smear microscopy
Xp= Xpert MTB/RIF

Prevalence	PPV
0.5%	75%
1%	86%
2%	93%

Prevalence	NPV
0.5%	99.7%
1%	99.5%
2%	98.9%

Prevalence	% true cases detected by Xp only	Proportion of those tested by Xp that go to CD	% true cases detected after Xp plus CD	PPV of Xp plus CD
0.5%	32%	5%	32%	70%
1%	32%	5%	32%	83%
2%	32%	20%	32%	85%

Algorithm 1c (chest X-ray available, Xpert MTB/RIF not available)

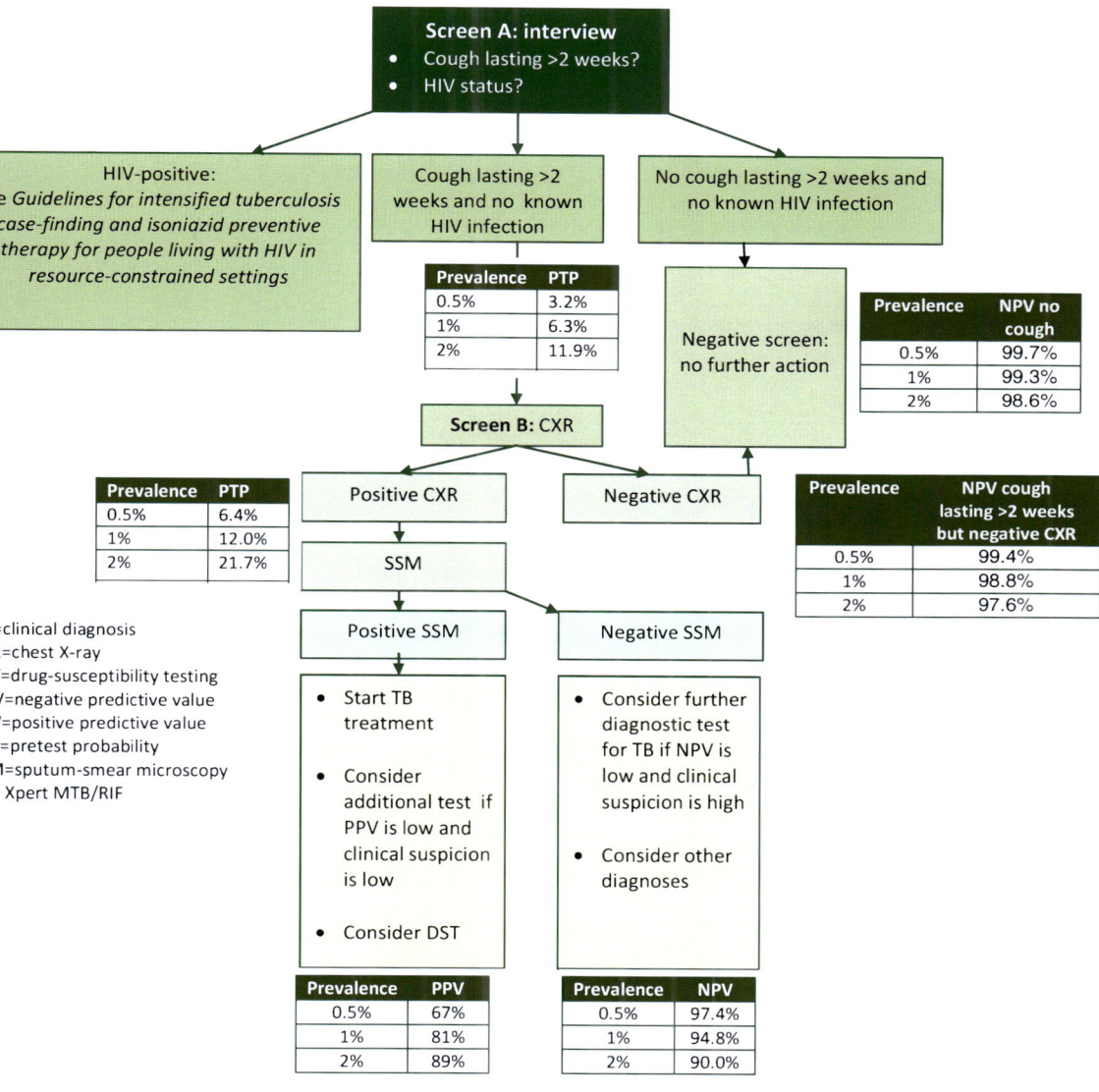

Screen A: interview
- Cough lasting >2 weeks?
- HIV status?

HIV-positive:
ee Guidelines for intensified tuberculosis case-finding and isoniazid preventive therapy for people living with HIV in resource-constrained settings

Cough lasting >2 weeks and no known HIV infection

No cough lasting >2 weeks and no known HIV infection

Prevalence	PTP
0.5%	3.2%
1%	6.3%
2%	11.9%

Negative screen: no further action

Prevalence	NPV no cough
0.5%	99.7%
1%	99.3%
2%	98.6%

Screen B: CXR

Prevalence	PTP
0.5%	6.4%
1%	12.0%
2%	21.7%

Positive CXR

Negative CXR

Prevalence	NPV cough lasting >2 weeks but negative CXR
0.5%	99.4%
1%	98.8%
2%	97.6%

SSM

=clinical diagnosis
R=chest X-ray
T=drug-susceptibility testing
V=negative predictive value
V=positive predictive value
?=pretest probability
M=sputum-smear microscopy
= Xpert MTB/RIF

Positive SSM

Negative SSM

- Start TB treatment
- Consider additional test if PPV is low and clinical suspicion is low
- Consider DST

- Consider further diagnostic test for TB if NPV is low and clinical suspicion is high
- Consider other diagnoses

Prevalence	PPV
0.5%	67%
1%	81%
2%	89%

Prevalence	NPV
0.5%	97.4%
1%	94.8%
2%	90.0%

Prevalence	% true cases detected by SSM only	Proportion of smear-negative that go to CD	% true cases detected after SSM plus CD	PPV SSM plus CD
0.5%	19%	100%	22%	38%
1%	19%	100%	22%	55%
2%	19%	100%	22%	72%

Algorithm 1d (chest X-ray and Xpert MTB/RIF available)

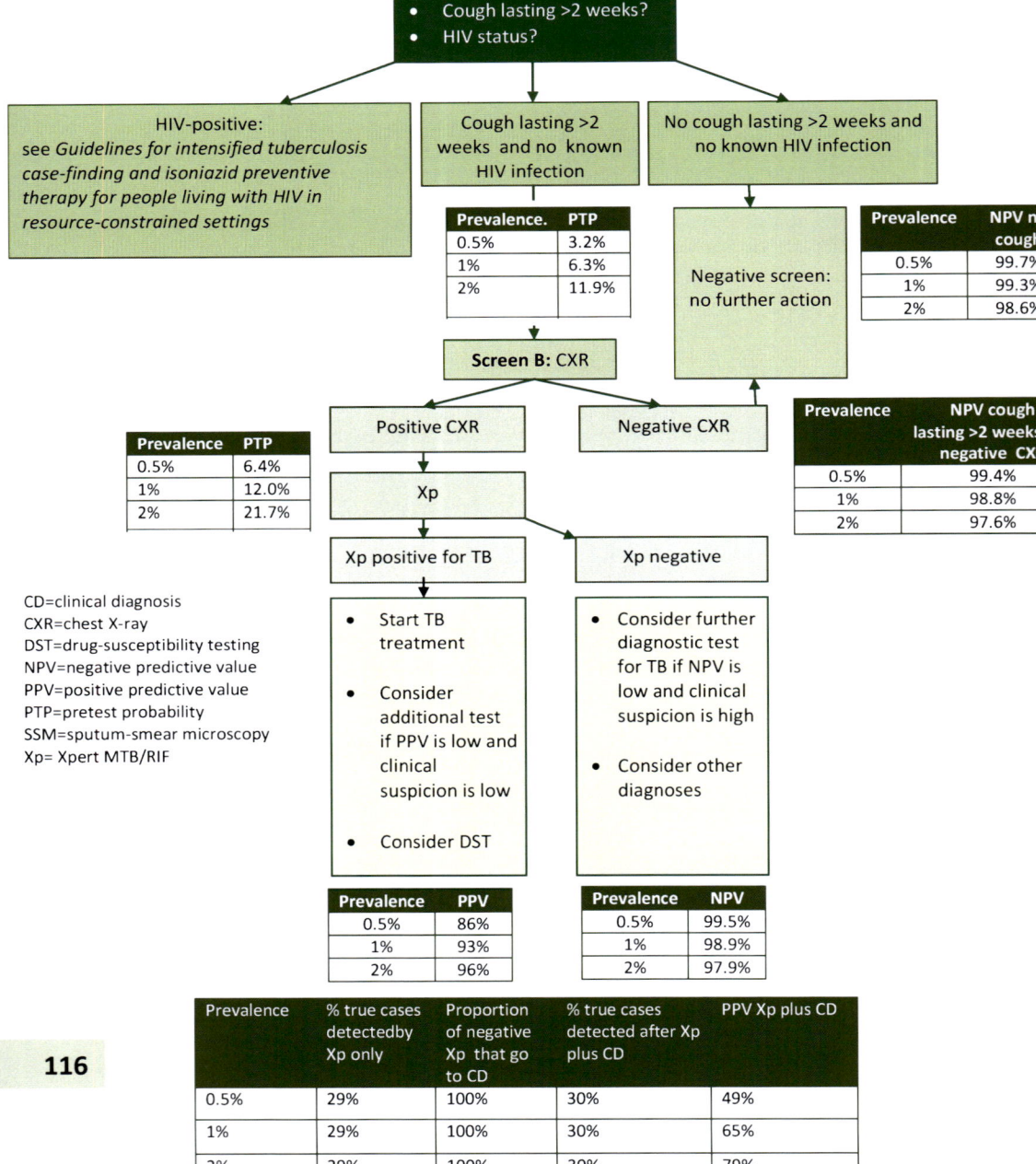

Algorithm 2a (chest X-ray and Xpert MTB/RIF not available)

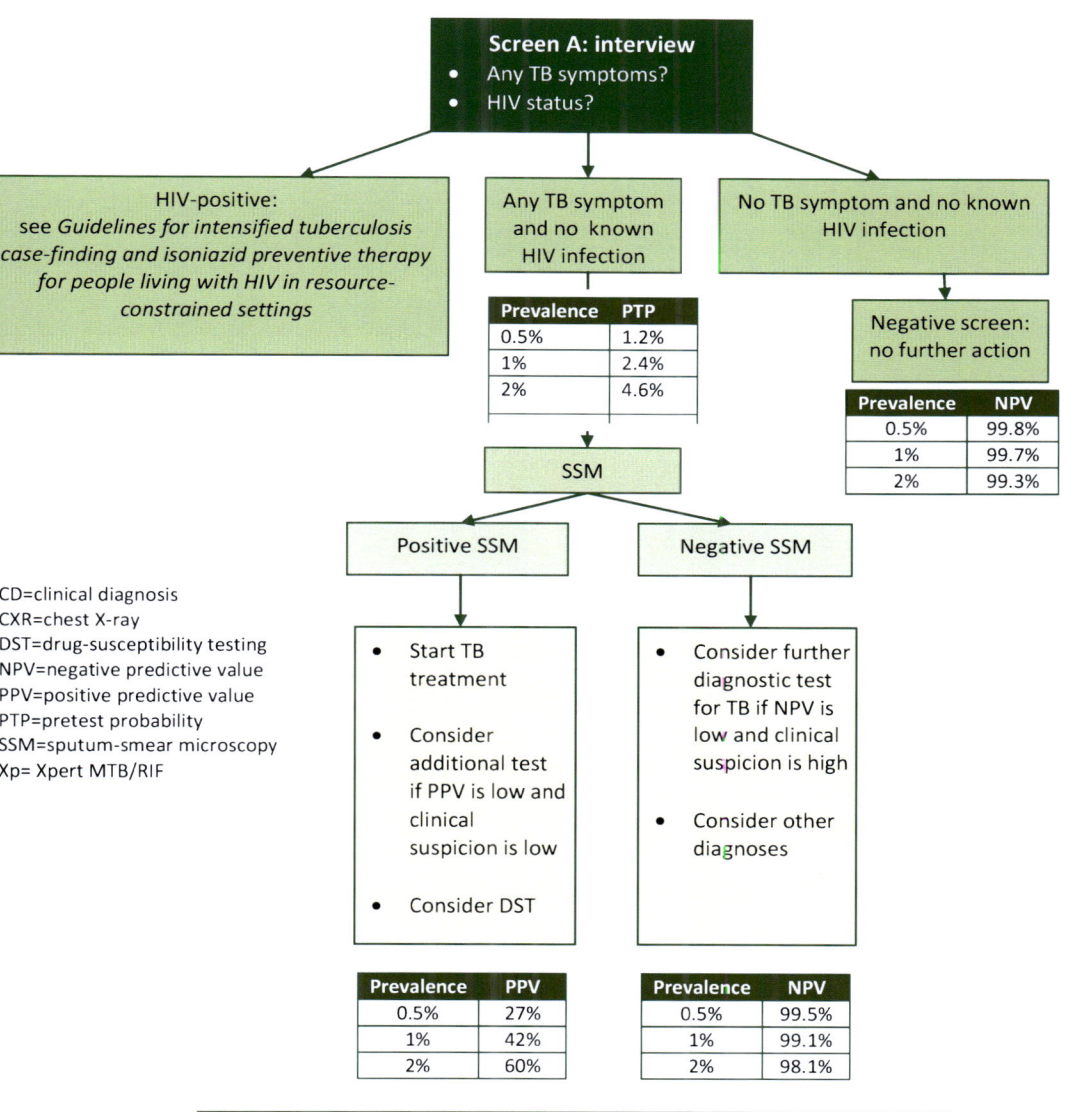

Screen A: interview
- Any TB symptoms?
- HIV status?

HIV-positive:
see *Guidelines for intensified tuberculosis case-finding and isoniazid preventive therapy for people living with HIV in resource-constrained settings*

Any TB symptom and no known HIV infection

Prevalence	PTP
0.5%	1.2%
1%	2.4%
2%	4.6%

No TB symptom and no known HIV infection

Negative screen: no further action

Prevalence	NPV
0.5%	99.8%
1%	99.7%
2%	99.3%

SSM

Positive SSM

CD=clinical diagnosis
CXR=chest X-ray
DST=drug-susceptibility testing
NPV=negative predictive value
PPV=positive predictive value
PTP=pretest probability
SSM=sputum-smear microscopy
Xp= Xpert MTB/RIF

- Start TB treatment
- Consider additional test if PPV is low and clinical suspicion is low
- Consider DST

Negative SSM

- Consider further diagnostic test for TB if NPV is low and clinical suspicion is high
- Consider other diagnoses

Prevalence	PPV
0.5%	27%
1%	42%
2%	60%

Prevalence	NPV
0.5%	99.5%
1%	99.1%
2%	98.1%

Prevalence	% true cases detected SSM only	Proportion of smear-negative that go to CD	% true cases detected after SSM and CD	PPV SSM plus CD
0.5%	47%	5%	47%	24%
1%	47%	10%	48%	37%
2%	47%	20%	48%	49%

117

Algorithm 2b (chest X-ray not available, Xpert MTB/RIF available)

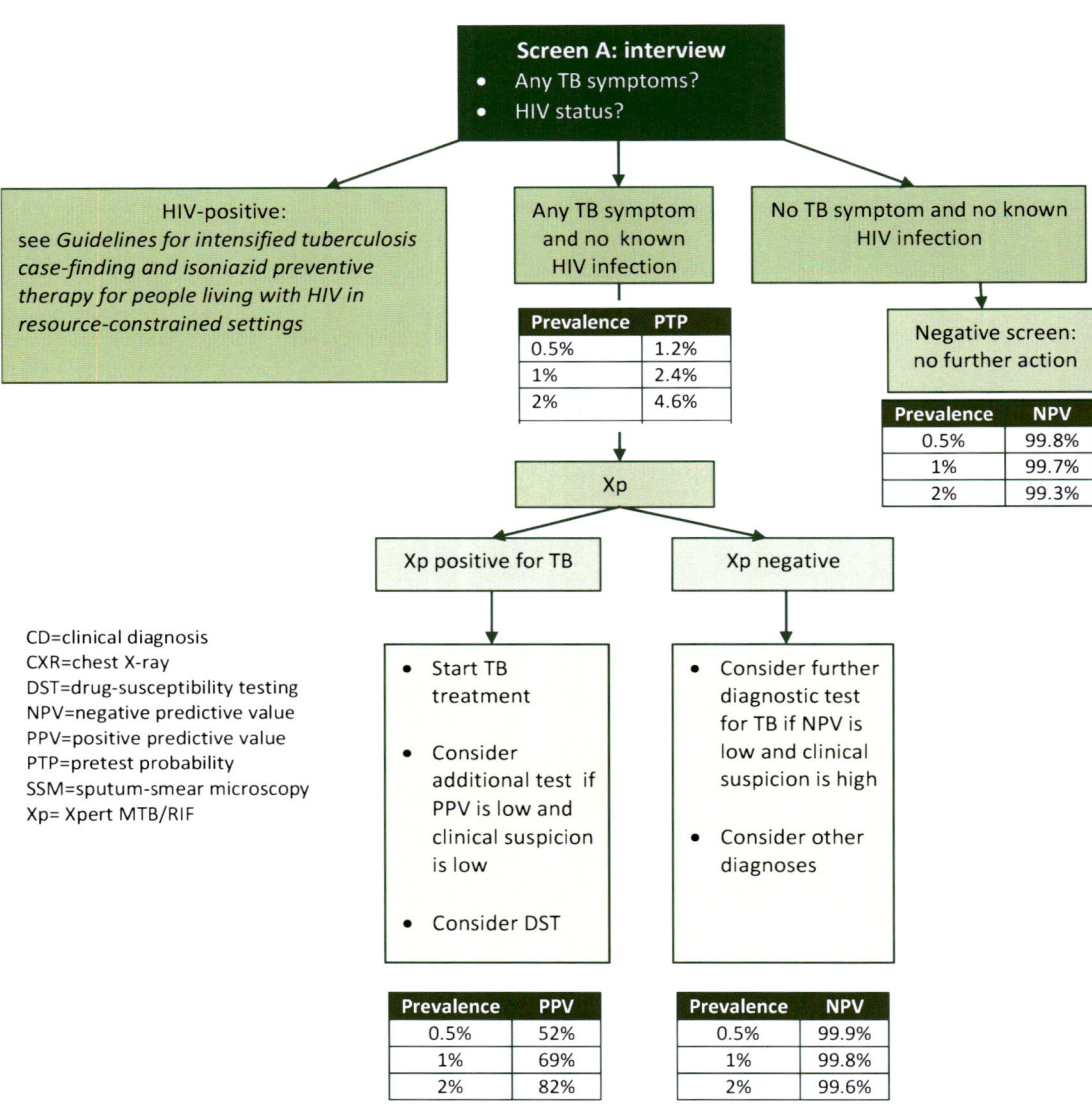

Screen A: interview
- Any TB symptoms?
- HIV status?

HIV-positive:
see *Guidelines for intensified tuberculosis case-finding and isoniazid preventive therapy for people living with HIV in resource-constrained settings*

Any TB symptom and no known HIV infection

Prevalence	PTP
0.5%	1.2%
1%	2.4%
2%	4.6%

No TB symptom and no known HIV infection

Negative screen: no further action

Prevalence	NPV
0.5%	99.8%
1%	99.7%
2%	99.3%

Xp

Xp positive for TB

Xp negative

CD=clinical diagnosis
CXR=chest X-ray
DST=drug-susceptibility testing
NPV=negative predictive value
PPV=positive predictive value
PTP=pretest probability
SSM=sputum-smear microscopy
Xp= Xpert MTB/RIF

- Start TB treatment
- Consider additional test if PPV is low and clinical suspicion is low
- Consider DST

- Consider further diagnostic test for TB if NPV is low and clinical suspicion is high
- Consider other diagnoses

Prevalence	PPV
0.5%	52%
1%	69%
2%	82%

Prevalence	NPV
0.5%	99.9%
1%	99.8%
2%	99.6%

Prevalence	% true cases detected Xp only	Proportion of negative Xp that go to CD	% true cases detected after Xp plus CD	PPV Xp plus CD
0.5%	71%	5%	71%	46%
1%	71%	5%	71%	63%
2%	71%	5%	71%	78%

Algorithm 2c (chest X-ray available, Xpert MTB/RIF not available)

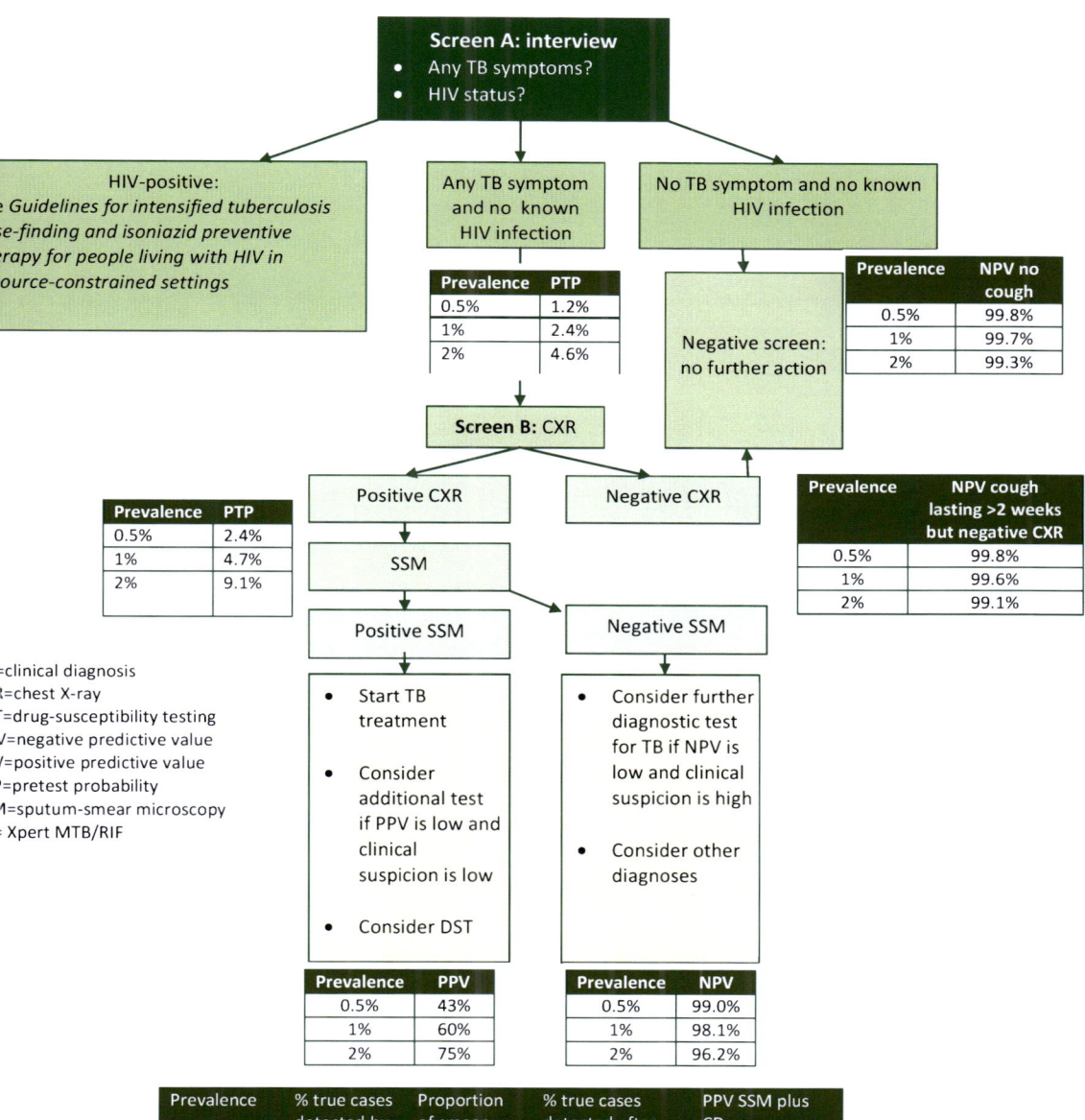

Screen A: interview
- Any TB symptoms?
- HIV status?

HIV-positive:
See Guidelines for intensified tuberculosis case-finding and isoniazid preventive therapy for people living with HIV in resource-constrained settings

Any TB symptom and no known HIV infection

Prevalence	PTP
0.5%	1.2%
1%	2.4%
2%	4.6%

No TB symptom and no known HIV infection

Negative screen: no further action

Prevalence	NPV no cough
0.5%	99.8%
1%	99.7%
2%	99.3%

Screen B: CXR

Prevalence	PTP
0.5%	2.4%
1%	4.7%
2%	9.1%

Positive CXR

Negative CXR

Prevalence	NPV cough lasting >2 weeks but negative CXR
0.5%	99.8%
1%	99.6%
2%	99.1%

SSM

Positive SSM

Negative SSM

CD=clinical diagnosis
CXR=chest X-ray
DST=drug-susceptibility testing
NPV=negative predictive value
PPV=positive predictive value
PTP=pretest probability
SSM=sputum-smear microscopy
X= Xpert MTB/RIF

Positive SSM
- Start TB treatment
- Consider additional test if PPV is low and clinical suspicion is low
- Consider DST

Negative SSM
- Consider further diagnostic test for TB if NPV is low and clinical suspicion is high
- Consider other diagnoses

Prevalence	PPV
0.5%	43%
1%	60%
2%	75%

Prevalence	NPV
0.5%	99.0%
1%	98.1%
2%	96.2%

Prevalence	% true cases detected by SSM only	Proportion of smear-negative that go to CD	% true cases detected after SSM plus CD	PPV SSM plus CD
0.5%	42%	10%	43%	37%
1%	42%	20%	44%	50%
2%	42%	40%	45%	60%

119

Algorithm 2d (chest X-ray and Xpert MTB/RIF available)

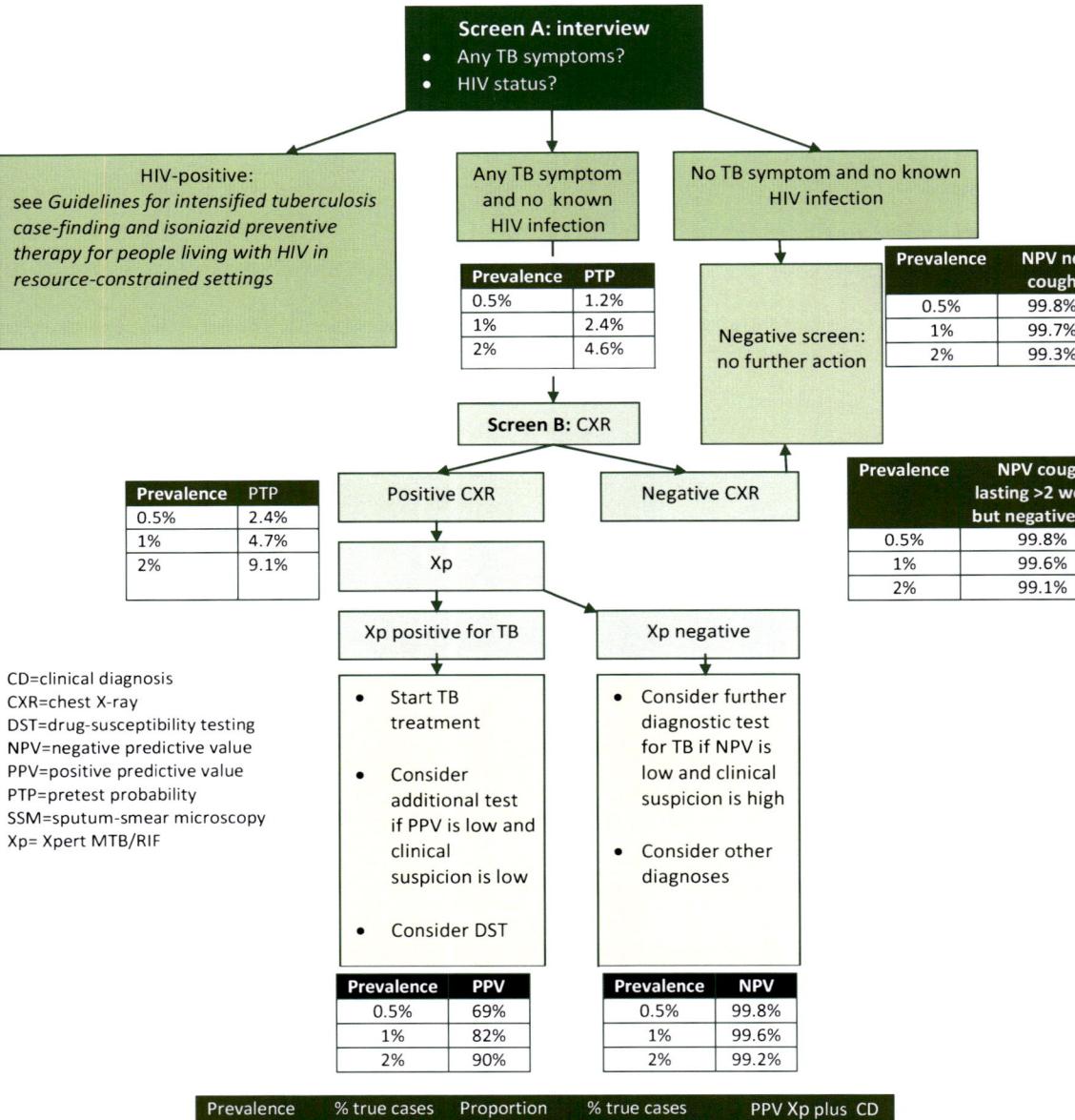

Screen A: interview
- Any TB symptoms?
- HIV status?

HIV-positive:
see *Guidelines for intensified tuberculosis case-finding and isoniazid preventive therapy for people living with HIV in resource-constrained settings*

Any TB symptom and no known HIV infection

Prevalence	PTP
0.5%	1.2%
1%	2.4%
2%	4.6%

No TB symptom and no known HIV infection

Prevalence	NPV no cough
0.5%	99.8%
1%	99.7%
2%	99.3%

Negative screen: no further action

Screen B: CXR

Prevalence	PTP
0.5%	2.4%
1%	4.7%
2%	9.1%

Positive CXR

Negative CXR

Prevalence	NPV cough lasting >2 weeks but negative CXR
0.5%	99.8%
1%	99.6%
2%	99.1%

Xp

Xp positive for TB

- Start TB treatment
- Consider additional test if PPV is low and clinical suspicion is low
- Consider DST

Xp negative

- Consider further diagnostic test for TB if NPV is low and clinical suspicion is high
- Consider other diagnoses

CD=clinical diagnosis
CXR=chest X-ray
DST=drug-susceptibility testing
NPV=negative predictive value
PPV=positive predictive value
PTP=pretest probability
SSM=sputum-smear microscopy
Xp= Xpert MTB/RIF

Prevalence	PPV
0.5%	69%
1%	82%
2%	90%

Prevalence	NPV
0.5%	99.8%
1%	99.6%
2%	99.2%

Prevalence	% true cases detected by Xp only	Proportion of negative Xp that go to CD	% true cases detected after Xp plus CD	PPV Xp plus CD
0.5%	64%	5%	64%	64%
1%	64%	5%	64%	78%
2%	64%	10%	64%	85%

Algorithm 3a (Xpert MTB/RIF not available)

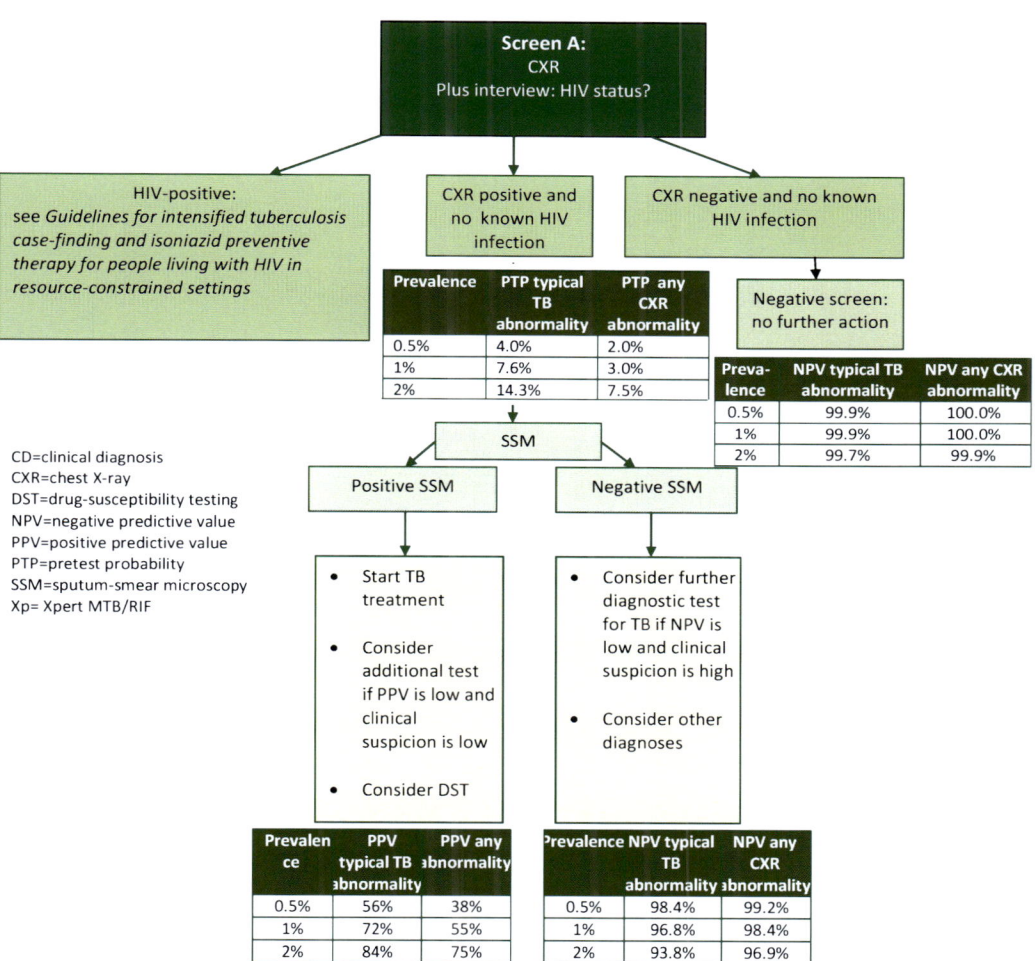

Screen A:
CXR
Plus interview: HIV status?

HIV-positive:
see *Guidelines for intensified tuberculosis case-finding and isoniazid preventive therapy for people living with HIV in resource-constrained settings*

CXR positive and no known HIV infection

CXR negative and no known HIV infection

Negative screen: no further action

Prevalence	PTP typical TB abnormality	PTP any CXR abnormality
0.5%	4.0%	2.0%
1%	7.6%	3.0%
2%	14.3%	7.5%

Preva-lence	NPV typical TB abnormality	NPV any CXR abnormality
0.5%	99.9%	100.0%
1%	99.9%	100.0%
2%	99.7%	99.9%

SSM

Positive SSM

Negative SSM

Positive SSM:
- Start TB treatment
- Consider additional test if PPV is low and clinical suspicion is low
- Consider DST

Negative SSM:
- Consider further diagnostic test for TB if NPV is low and clinical suspicion is high
- Consider other diagnoses

CD=clinical diagnosis
CXR=chest X-ray
DST=drug-susceptibility testing
NPV=negative predictive value
PPV=positive predictive value
PTP=pretest probability
SSM=sputum-smear microscopy
Xp= Xpert MTB/RIF

Prevalence	PPV typical TB abnormality	PPV any abnormality
0.5%	56%	38%
1%	72%	55%
2%	84%	75%

Prevalence	NPV typical TB abnormality	NPV any CXR abnormality
0.5%	98.4%	99.2%
1%	96.8%	98.4%
2%	93.8%	96.9%

Preva-lence	Typical CXR abnormality suggestive of active TB				Any CXR abnormality suggestive of active or inactive TB			
	% true cases detected by SSM only	Proportion of smear-negative that go to CD	% true cases detected by SSM plus CD	PPV SSM plus CD	% true cases detected by SSM only	Proportion of smear-negative that go to CD	% true cases detected by SSM plus CD	PPV SSM plus CD
0.5%	53%	20%	55%	45%	60%	10%	61%	32%
1%	53%	40%	56%	56%	60%	20%	61%	45%
2%	53%	70%	59%	65%	60%	40%	63%	55%

Algorithm 3b (Xpert MTB/RIF available)

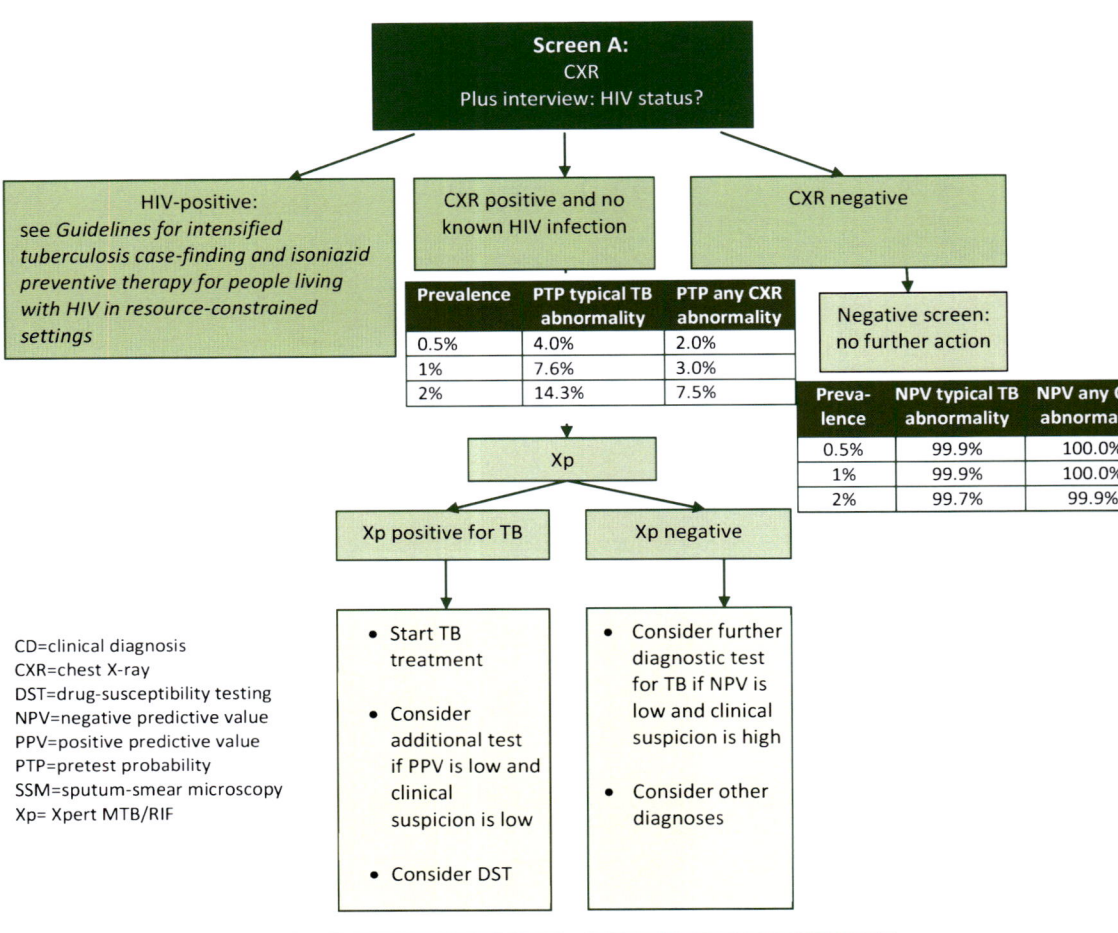

Screen A:
CXR
Plus interview: HIV status?

HIV-positive:
see *Guidelines for intensified tuberculosis case-finding and isoniazid preventive therapy for people living with HIV in resource-constrained settings*

CXR positive and no known HIV infection

Prevalence	PTP typical TB abnormality	PTP any CXR abnormality
0.5%	4.0%	2.0%
1%	7.6%	3.0%
2%	14.3%	7.5%

CXR negative

Negative screen: no further action

Preva-lence	NPV typical TB abnormality	NPV any CXR abnormality
0.5%	99.9%	100.0%
1%	99.9%	100.0%
2%	99.7%	99.9%

Xp

Xp positive for TB

Xp negative

CD=clinical diagnosis
CXR=chest X-ray
DST=drug-susceptibility testing
NPV=negative predictive value
PPV=positive predictive value
PTP=pretest probability
SSM=sputum-smear microscopy
Xp= Xpert MTB/RIF

- Start TB treatment
- Consider additional test if PPV is low and clinical suspicion is low
- Consider DST

- Consider further diagnostic test for TB if NPV is low and clinical suspicion is high
- Consider other diagnoses

Preva-lence	PPV typical TB abnormality	PPV any abnormality
0.5%	79%	65%
1%	88%	79%
2%	94%	88%

Preva-lence	NPV typical TB abnormality	NPV any abnormality
0.5%	99.7%	99.8%
1%	99.4%	99.7%
2%	98.7%	99.4%

Preva-lence	Typical CXR abnormality suggestive of active TB				Any CXR abnormality suggestive of active or inactive TB			
	% true cases detected by Xp only	Proportion of negative Xp that go to CD	% true cases detected by Xp plus CD	PPV Xp plus CD	% true cases detected by Xp only	Proportion of negative Xp that go to CD	% true cases detected by Xp plus CD	PPV Xp plus CD
0.5%	80%	5%	80%	75%	90%	5%	90%	59%
1%	80%	10%	80%	83%	90%	5%	90%	74%
2%	80%	20%	80%	88%	90%	10%	90%	83%

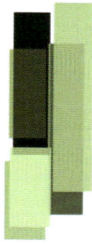

Annex IV.
Guideline Development Group, WHO secretariat and peer reviewers

Guideline Development Group

Dr Sevim Ahmedov
Senior TB Technical Adviser, United States Agency for International Development, USA

Dr Helen Ayles
Researcher, University of Zambia, Zambia

Dr Lucie Blok
Senior Adviser, Health, KIT Development Policy and Practice, KIT Royal Tropical Institute, the Netherlands

Dr Gavin Churchyard
Chief Executive Officer, Aurum Institute for Health Research, South Africa

Dr Liz Corbett
Reader in Infectious and Tropical Diseases, London School of Tropical Medicine and Hygiene and MLW Clinical Research Programme, Malawi

Dr Mao Tang Eang
Manager, National TB Programme, Cambodia

Dr Peter Godfrey-Faussett
Researcher, London School of Hygiene and Tropical Medicine, United Kingdom

Dr Jonathan Golub
Researcher., Johns Hopkins University School of Medicine, United States

Dr Katharina Kranzer
Researcher, London School of Hygiene and Tropical Medicine, United Kingdom

Dr Josué Lima
National TB Programme, Brazil

Dr Wang Lixia
Manager, National TB Programme, People's Republic of China

Dr Thandar Lwin
Manager, National TB Programme, Myanmar

Dr Ellen Mitchell
Senior Epidemiologist, KNCV Tuberculosis Foundation, the Netherlands

Dr Mary Reichler
Medical epidemiologist, Division of TB Elimination, Centers for Disease Control and Prevention, USA

Dr Adrienne Shapiro
Researcher, John Hopkins University School of Medicine, USA

Dr David Sinclair
Guideline methodologist. Effective Health Care RPC, Cochrane Infectious Diseases Group, Liverpool School of Tropical Medicine, United Kingdom

Dr Alena Skrahina
Deputy Manager, National TB Programme, Belarus

Dr Pedro Guillermo Suarez
Management Science for Health (MSH), USA

Dr Marieke van der Werf
Head, TB Programme, European Centre for Disease Prevention and Control, Sweden

Dr Anja Van't Hoog
Researcher, Amsterdam Institute for Global Health ard Development, the Netherlands

Dr Norio Yamada
Director, Department of International Cooperation, Research Institute for TB (RIT), Japan Anti-TB Association (JATA), Japan

WHO Secretariat
Mr Jacob Creswell, The Stop TB Partnership secretariat
Dr Leopold Blanc, Stop TB Department
Dr Daniel Chemtob, Stop TB Department
Dr Haileyesus Getahun, Stop TB Department
Dr Philippe Glaziou, Stop TB Department
Dr Malgosia Grzemska, Stop TB Department
Dr Dennis Falzon, Stop TB Department
Dr Ernesto Jaramillo, Stop TB Department
Dr Daniel Kibuga, Regional Office for Africa
Dr Knut Lönnroth, Stop TB Department
Dr Ikushi Onozaki, Stop TB Department
Dr Salah Ottmani, Stop TB Department
Dr Mario Raviglione, Stop TB Department
Dr Andreas Reis, Department for Ethics, Equity, Trade and Human Rights
Dr Suvanand Sahu, the Stop TB Partnership secretariat
Dr Mukund Uplekar, Stop TB Department
Mr Wayne Van Gemert, Stop TB Department
Dr Catharina van Weezenbeek, Regional Office for the Western Pacific
Ms Diana Weil, Coordinator, Stop TB Department
Dr Karin Weyer, Coordinator, Stop TB Department

Peer reviewers
Dr Martien Borgdorff, University of Amsterdam, the Netherlands
Dr Frank Cobelens, Amsterdam Institute for Global Health and Development, the Netherlands
Dr Paul Douglas, Department of Immigration and Citizenship, Australia
Dr Steven Graham, Childhood TB Subgroup, Centre for International Child Health, Australia

Dr Anthony D Harries, International Union Against Tuberculosis and Lung Disease, United Kingdom
Dr Giovanni B Migliori, European Respiratory Society, WHO Collaborating Centre for TB and Lung Diseases, Italy
Dr Lisa Nelson, WHO, HIV Department
Dr Alasdair Reid, UNAIDS, South Africa

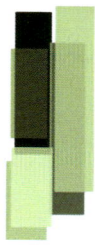

References

[1] Lozano R, et al. Global and regional mortality from 235 causes of death for 20 age groups in 1990 and 2010: a systematic analysis for the Global Burden of Disease Study 2010. *Lancet*, 2012, 380:2095–2128.

[2] Murray CJL et al. Disability-adjusted life years (DALYs) for 291 diseases and injuries in 21 regions, 1990–2010: a systematic analysis for the Global Burden of Disease Study 2010. *Lancet,* 2012, 380:2197–2223.

[3] *Global tuberculosis control 2011*. Geneva, World Health Organization, 2012.

[4] *WHO Expert Committee on Tuberculosis: ninth report*. Geneva, World Health Organization, 1974:16   (WHO Technical Report Series, No. 552).

[5] Meijer J et al. Identification of sources of infection. *Bulletin of the International Union Against Tuberculosis*, 1971, 45:5-54.

[6] Rieder H. What is the role of case detection by periodic mass radiographic examination in TB control? In: Frieden T, ed. *Toman's tuberculosis*, 2nd ed. Geneva, World Health Organization, 2004:72–79.

[7] Krivinka R et al.. Epidemiological and clinical study of tuberculosis in the district of Kolin, Czechoslovakia: sSecond report (1965-1972). *Bulletin of the World Health Organization,* 1974, 51:59-69.

[8] Roelsgaard E, Iversen E, Bløcher C. Tuberculosis in tropical Africa – an epidemiological study. *Bulletin of the World Health Organization,* 1964, 30:459–518.

[9] *WHO Expert Committee on Tuberculosis: eighth report*. Geneva, World Health Organization, 1964 (WHO Technical Report Series, No. 290).

[10] *Guidelines for intensified tuberculosis case-finding and isoniazid preventive therapy for people living with HIV in resource-constrained settings*. Geneva, World Health Organization, 2011. (WHO/HTM/TB/2011.11)

[11] *Recommendations for investigating the contacts of persons with infectious tuberculosis in low- and middle-income countries*. Geneva, World Health Organization, 2012 (WHO/HTM/TB/2012.9).

[12] *Guidelines for the control of tuberculosis in prisons*. The Hague, Tuberculosis Coalition for Technical Assistance (TBCTA), 2009.

[13] *Tuberculosis care and control in refugee and displaced populations: an interagency field manual*, 2nd ed. Geneva, World Health Organization, 2007 (WHO/HTM/TB/2007.377.).

[14] *Collaborative framework for care and control of tuberculosis and diabetes*. Geneva, World Health Organization, 2011 (WHO/HTM/TB/2011.15).

[15] Broekmans JF et al. European framework for tuberculosis control and elimination in countries with a low incidence: recommendations of the World Health Organization (WHO), International Union Against Tuberculosis and Lung Disease

(IUATLD) and Royal Netherlands Tuberculosis Association (KNCV) Working Group. *European Respiratory Journal,* 2002, 19:765–775.

[16] *Guidelines for the programmatic management of drug-resistant tuberculosis: 2011 update.* Geneva, World Health Organization, 2011 (WHO/HTM/TB/2011.6).

[17] *Policy guidelines for collaborative TB and HIV services for injecting and other drug users: an integrated approach.* Geneva, World Health Organization, 2008 (WHO/HTM/TB/2008.404).

[18] Golub JE et al. Active case finding of tuberculosis: historical perspective and future prospects. *International Journal of Tuberculosis and Lung Disease,* 2005, 9:1183–1203.

[19] *Tuberculosis control in high risk groups inn the Netherlands.* The Hague: KNCV, 1997.

[20] Raviglione M et al. Scaling up interventions to achieve global tuberculosis control: progress and new developments. *Lancet* 2012, 379:1902–1913.

[21] Luelmo F. What is the role of case detection in tuberculosis control. In: Frieden T, ed. *Toman's tuberculosis,* 2nd ed. Geneva, WHO, 2004: 3–5.

[22] Lin X et al. Dose–response relationship between treatment delay of smear-positive tuberculosis patients and intra-household transmission: a cross-sectional study. *Transactions of the Royal Society of Tropical Medicine and Hygiene,* 2008, 102:797-804.

[23] Lönnroth K et al. Tuberculosis control and elimination 2010-50: cure, care, and social development. *Lancet.* 2010, 375:1814–1829.

[24] Lönnroth K et al. Drivers of tuberculosis epidemics: the role of risk factors and social determinants. *Social Science and Medicine,* 2009, 68 :2240–2246.

[25] Storla DG, Yimer S, Bjune GA. A systematic review of delay in the diagnosis and treatment of tuberculosis. *BMC Public Health* 2008, 8:15 (doi: 10.1186/1471-2458-8-15).

[26] Sreeramareddy CT, et al. Time delays in diagnosis of pulmonary tuberculosis: a systematic review of literature. *BMC Infectious Diseases* 2009, 9:91 (doi:10.1186/1471-2334-9-91).

[27] Hoa NB et al. A national survey of tuberculosis prevalence in Vietnam. *Bulletin of the World Health Organization,* 2010, 88:273–280.

[28] *National TB Prevalence Survey, 2002, Cambodia.* Phnom Penh: Ministry of Health, 2002.

[29] Ayles H et al. Prevalence of tuberculosis, HIV and respiratory symptoms in two Zambian communities: implications for tuberculosis control in the era of HIV. *PLoS One* 2009, 4:e5602 (doi:10.1371/journal.pone.0005602).

[30] Shapiro et al. *A systematic review of active case-finding strategies in risk groups for tuberculosis (TB) and the relationship to the number needed to screen: report to WHO.* Geneva, World Health Organization, 2012 (systematic review No 3 at www.who.int/tb/tbscreening).

[31] Getahun H et al. Development of a standardized screening rule for tuberculosis in people living with HIV in resource-constrained settings: individual participant data meta-analysis of observational studies. *PLoS Medicine,* 2011, 8(1):e1000391 (doi:10.1371/journal.pmed.1000391).

[32] Morrison J, Pai M, Hopewell PC. Tuberculosis and latent tuberculosis infection in close contacts of people with pulmonary tuberculosis in low-income and middle-income countries: a systematic review and meta-analysis. *Lancet Infectious Diseases,* 2008, 8:359–368.

[33] Fox GJ et al. Contact investigation for tuberculosis: a systematic review and meta-analysis. *European Respiratory Journal,* 2013, 41:140–156 (doi: 10.1183/09031936.00070812).

[34] Barboza CEG et al. Tuberculosis and silicosis: epidemiology, diagnosis and chemotherapy. *Jornal Brasileiro de Pneumologia,* 2008, 34:959–966.

[35] Baussano I et al. Tuberculosis incidence in prisons: a systematic review. *PLoS Medicine,* 2010, 7:e1000381 (doi:10.1371/journal.pmed.1000381).

[36] Beijer U, Wolf A, Fazel S. Prevalence of tuberculosis, hepatitis C virus, and HIV in homeless people: a systematic review and meta-analysis. *Lancet Infectious Diseases*, 2012, 12:859–870.

[37] *Global tuberculosis control 2011*. Geneva, World Health Organization, 2012.

[38] *Guidance for national tuberculosis programmes on the management of tuberculosis in children*. Geneva, World Health Organization, 2006 (WHO/HTM/TB/2006.371).

[39] Rutherford ME et al. Preventive therapy in children exposed to Mycobacterium tuberculosis: problems and solutions. *Tropical Medicine and International Health,* 2012, 17:1264–1273.

[40] *Implementing the WHO Stop TB Strategy: a handbook for national tuberculosis programmes*. Geneva, World Health Organization, 2008 (WHO/HTM/TB/2008.401).

[41] China Centre for Disease Control. [*The 5th National Tuberculosis Prevalence Survey in China – 2010.*] Beijing, Ministry of Health, 2011 [in Chinese].

[42] Behr MA et al. Transmission of Mycobacterium tuberculosis from patients smear-negative for acid-fast bacilli. *Lancet* 1999, 353:444–449.

[43] Tostmann A et al. Tuberculosis transmission by patients with smear-negative pulmonary tuberculosis in a large cohort in the Netherlands. *Clinical Infectious Diseases*, 2008, 47:1135–1142.

[44] Dowdy D, Chaisson R. The persistence of tuberculosis in the age of DOTS: reassessing the effect of case detection. *Bulletin of the World Health Organization,* 2009, 87:296–304.

[45] *Early detection of tuberculosis: an overview of approaches, guidelines and tools*. Geneva, World Health Organization, 2011 (WHO/HTM/STB/PSI/2011.21).

[46] *Scoping meeting for the development of guidelines on screening for active TB, 31 May – 1 June 2011.*Geneva, World Health Organization, 2011 (http://www.who.int/tb/guidlinesscreeningtb/en/index.html).

[47] Whiting PF et al. QUADAS-2: a revised tool for the quality assessment of diagnostic accuracy studies. *Annals of Internal Medicine*, 2011, 155:529–536.

[48] Reitsma JB et al. Assessing methodological quality. In: Deeks JJ, ed. *Cochrane handbook for systematic reviews of diagnostic test accuracy*. London, Cochrane Collaboration, 2009.

[49] *Automated real-time nucleic acid amplification technology for rapid and simultaneous detection of tuberculosis and rifampicin resistance: Xpert MTB/RIF system. Policy statement.* Geneva, World Health Organization, 2011 (WHO/HTM/TB/2011.4).

[50] *Approaches to improve sputum smear microscopy for tuberculosis diagnosis: expert group meeting report.* Geneva, World Health Organization, 2009.

[51] Cattamanchi A et al. Does bleach processing increase the accuracy of sputum smear microscopy for diagnosing pulmonary tuberculosis. *Journal of Clinical Microbiology,* 2010, 48:2433–2439.

[52] Vassal A, et al. Rapid diagnosis of tuberculosis with the Xpert MTB/RIF assay in high burden countries: a cost-effectiveness analysis. *PLoS Medicine,* 2011, 8(11):e1001120 (doi:10.1371/journal.pmed.1001120).

[53] Kruk A, Gie R, Schaaf S, Marias B. Symptom-based screening of child tuberculosis contacts: improved feasibility in resource-constrained settings. *Pediatrics,* 2008, 121;e1645–1652 (doi: 10.1542/peds.2007-3138).

[54] Song R et al. *Evaluation of tuberculosis screening approaches among HIV-infected children in Rwanda, 2008* [Abstract no. TUPEB132]. Geneva, International AIDS Society, 2013 (http://www.iasociety.org/Abstracts/A200721790.aspx, accessed 24.08.2012)

[55] Keown T, ed. *Screening in medical care: reviewing the evidence.* Oxford, Oxford University Press, 1968.

[56] Holland WW, Stewart S. *Screening in disease prevention: what works?* Milton Keynes, England, Radcliffe Health, 2005.

[57] Kranzer K et al. A systematic literature review of the benefits to communities and individuals of active screening for tuberculosis disease. *International Journal of Tuberculosis and Lung Disease,* 2013, 17:432–446. www.who.int/tb/tbscreening

[58] Murray CJL, Salomon JA. Modeling the impact of global tuberculosis control strategies. *Proceedings of the National Academy* of Sciences of the USA, 1998, 95:13881–13886.

[59] Borgdorff MW, Floyd K, Broekmans J. Interventions to reduce tuberculosis mortality and transmission in low- and middle-income countries. *Bulletin of the World Health Organization,* 2002, 80:217–227.

[60] Dodd PJ, Whit RG, Corbett EL. Periodic active case finding for TB: when to look? *PLoS One*, 2011, 6(12):e29130 (doi: 10.1371/journal.pone.0029130).

[61] Dowdy D et al. Heterogeneity in tuberculosis transmission and the role of geographic hotspots in propagating epidemics. *Proceedings of the National Academy of Sciences of the USA,* 2012, 109:9557–9562.

[62] Legrand J et al. Modeling the impact of tuberculosis control strategies in highly endemic overcrowded prisons. *PLoS One,* 2008, 3(5):e2100 (doi:10.1371/journal.pone.0002100).

[63] Tiemersma EW et al. Natural history of tuberculosis: duration and fatality of untreated pulmonary tuberculosis in HIV negative patients: a systematic review. *PLoS ONE,* 6(4):e17601 (doi:10.1371/journal.pone.0017601).

[64] Straetemans M et al. Assessing tuberculosis case fatality ratio: a meta-analysis. *PLoS One,* 6(6): e20755 (doi:10.1371/journal.pone.0020755).

[65] Waitt CJ, Squire SB. A systematic review of risk factors for death in adults during and after tuberculosis treatment. *International Journal of Tuberculosis and Lung Disease,* 2011,15:871–885.

[66] Miller TL et al. Personal and societal health quality lost to tuberculosis. *PLoS One* 2009, 4 :e5080 (doi:10.1371/journal.pone.0005080).

[67] Rieder H. *Epidemiological basis of tuberculosis control*. Paris, International Union Against Tuberculosis and Lung Disease, 1999.

[68] Frieden T. *Toman's tuberculosis,* 2nd ed. Geneva, World Health Organization, 2004.

[69] van't Hoog AH et al. *A systematic review of the sensitivity and specificity of symptoms and chest radiography as screening tools for active pulmonary tuberculosis: report to WHO*. Geneva, World Health Organization, 2012. www.who.int/tb/tbscreening.

[70] Mitchell E et al. *Acceptability of TB screening among at-risk and vulnerable groups: a systematic qualitative/quantitative literature metasynthesis: report to WHO.* Geneva, World Health Organization, 2012. Mitchell E et al. *Acceptability of household and community-based TB screening in high burden communities: A systematic literature review: report to WHO.* Geneva, World Health Organization, 2012. www.who.int/tb/tbscreening

[71] Hopewell PC et al. International standards for tuberculosis care. *Lancet Infectious Diseases, 2006*, 6:710–725.

[72] *Guidance for national tuberculosis programmes on the management of tuberculosis in children*, 2nd ed.. Geneva, World Health Organization, 2013.

[73] *Guideline: nutritional care and support for patients with tuberculosis.* Geneva, World Health Organization, 2013.

[74] *Rapid implementation of the Xpert MTB/RIF diagnostic test: technical and operational 'how-to'. Practical considerations.* Geneva, World Health Organization, 2011 (WHO/HTM/TB/2011.2).

[75] *WHO policy on collaborative TB/HIV activities: guidelines for national programmes and other stakeholders.* Geneva, World Health Organization. 2012 (WHO/HTM/TB/2012.1).

[76] *WHO policy on TB infection control in health-care facilities, congregate settings and households.* Geneva, World Health Organization, 2009 (WHO/HTM/TB/2009.419).

[77] *Implementing the WHO Stop TB Strategy: a handbook for national tuberculosis control programmes*. Geneva, World Health Organization, 2008 (WHO/HTM/TB/2008.401).

[78] Lönnroth K et al. A homogeneous dose-response relationship between body-mass index and tuberculosis incidence. *International Journal of Epidemiology*, 2009, 9:149–155.

[79] Cegielski, JP, McMurray DN. The relationship between malnutrition and tuberculosis: evidence from studies in humans and experimental animals. *International Journal of Tuberculosis and Lung Disease*, 2004, 8:286–298.

[80] Targeted tuberculin testing and treatment of latent tuberculosis infection. *Morbidity and Mortality Weekly Report: Recommendations and Reports, 2000*, 49(RR 6):1–51.

[81] Jeon CY, Murray MB. Diabetes mellitus increases the risk of active tuberculosis: a systematic review of 13 observational studies. *PLoS Medicine, 2008*, 5:e152 (doi:10.1371/journal.pmed.0050152).

[82] Baker MA et al. The impact of diabetes on tuberculosis treatment outcomes: a systematic review. *BMC Medicine*, 2011 9:81 (doi:10.1186/1741-7015-9-81).

[83] Lönnroth K et al. Alcohol use as a risk factor for tuberculosis – a systematic review. *BMC Public Health*, 2008, 8:289 (doi:10.1186/1471-2458/8/289).

[84] Rehm J et al. The association between alcohol use, alcohol use disorders and tuberculosis (TB). A systematic review. *BMC Public Health* 2009, 9:450 (doi:10.1186/1471-2458-9-450).

[85] Lin H, Ezzati M, Murray M. Tobacco smoke, indoor air pollution and tuberculosis: a systematic review and meta-analysis. *PLoS Medicine*, 2007, 4(1): e20 (doi:10.1371/journal.pmed.0040020).

[86] Slama K et al. Tobacco and tuberculosis: a qualitative systematic review and meta analysis. *International Journal of Tuberculosis and Lung Disease*, 2007, 11:1049–1061.

[87] Verver S, Warren RM, Beyers N. Rate of reinfection tuberculosis after successful treatment is higher than rate of new tuberculosis. *American Journal of Respiratory and Critical Care Medicine*, 2005, 171:1430–1435.

[88] Crampina AC et al. Recurrent TB: relapse or reinfection? The effect of HIV in a general population cohort in Malawi. *AIDS* 2010, 24:417–426.

[89] Marx FM et al. The rate of sputum smear-positive tuberculosis after treatment default in a high-burden setting: a retrospective cohort study. *PLoS One*, 2012, 7(9):e45724 (doi:10.1371/journal.pone.0045724).

[90] Getahun H et al. Prevention, diagnosis, and treatment of tuberculosis in children and mothers: evidence for action for maternal, neonatal, and child health services. *Journal of Infectious Diseases*, 2012, 205(Suppl.):S216–S227.

[91] Figueroa-Damian R, Arredondo-Garcia JL. Neonatal outcome of children born to women with tuberculosis. *Archives of Medical Research*, 2001, 32:66–69.

[92] Jana N et al. Perinatal outcome in pregnancies complicated by pulmonary tuberculosis. *International Journal of Gynaecology and Obstetrics*, 1994, 44:119–124.

[93] Asuquo J et al. A case-control study of the risk of adverse perinatal outcomes due to tuberculosis during pregnancy. *Obstetrics and Gynecology,* 2012, 32:635–638.

[94] Jana N et al. Obstetrical outcomes among women with extrapulmonary tuberculosis. *New England Journal of Medicine,* 1999; 341:645–649.

[95] Kothari A, Mahadevan N, Girling J. Tuberculosis and pregnancy – results of a study in a high prevalence area in London. *European Journal of Obstetrics, Gynecology and Reproductive Biology,* 2006, 126:48–55.

[96] Heywood S et al. A survey of pregnant women with tuberculosis at the Port Moresby General Hospital. *Papua and New Guinea Medical Journal,* 1999, 42:63-70.

[97] Bjerkedal T, Bahna SL, Lehmann EH. Course and outcome of pregnancy in women with pulmonary tuberculosis. *Scandinavian Journal of Respiratory Diseases,* 1975, 56:245–50.

[98] Nhan-Chang CL, Jones TB. Tuberculosis in pregnancy. *Clinical Obstetrics and Gynecology,* 2010, 53:311–321.

[99] *Tuberculosis prevalence surveys: a handbook.* Geneva, World Health Organization, 2011 (WHO/HTM/TB/2010.17).

[100] *Practical approach to lung health (PAL): a primary health care strategy for the integrated management of respiratory conditions in people of five years of age and over.* Geneva, World Health Organization, 2005 (WHO/HTM/TB/2005.351; WHO/NMH/CHP/CPM/CRA/05.3).

[101] *A WHO/The Union monograph on TB and tobacco control: joining efforts to control two related global epidemics.* Geneva, World Health Organization, 2008 (WHO/TB/2007.390).

[102] Dara M et al. The history and evolution of immigration medical screening for tuberculosis. *Expert Review of Anti-infective Therapy,* 2013, 11:137–146.

[103] Cuevas LE et al. LED fluorescence microscopy for the diagnosis of pulmonary tuberculosis: a multi-country cross-sectional evaluation. *PLoS Medicine,* 2011, 8(7):e1001057 (doi:10.1371/journal.pmed.1001057).